'Martin-Sperry's book *Couples and Sex* is a readable explanation of the factors that co have sexual difficulty. It makes clear to the clinician why sex occur, and shows how to understand and help with these problems. Since sexual difficulties are central to the distress that brings so many couples to counseling or therapy, this is crucial information that is, however, rarely taught in clinical training programs. This slim volume gives the therapist the basics she needs to know, and at the same time serves as a ready reference for the experienced clinician. I recommend this book to both experienced and new therapists, and to all clinicians who want to know more about the crucial role of sex in couple relationships.'

David E Scharff MD
Co-Director
International Institute of Object Relations Therapy (IIORT)
Washington, DC, USA

Couples and Sex

An introduction to relationship dynamics and psychosexual concepts

Carol Martin-Sperry
Couples and Psychosexual Therapist

Foreword by
Christopher Clulow
Director, The Tavistock Marital Studies Institute

Radcliffe Medical Press

Radcliffe Medical Press Ltd
18 Marcham Road
Abingdon
Oxon OX14 1AA
United Kingdom

www.radcliffe-oxford.com
The Radcliffe Medical Press electronic catalogue and online ordering facility.
Direct sales to anywhere in the world.

British Library Cataloguing in Publication Data

A catalogue record for this book is available from the British Library.

ISBN 1 85775 816 1

Typeset by Advance Typesetting Ltd, Oxfordshire
Printed and bound by TJ International Ltd, Padstow, Cornwall

Contents

Foreword

Sex permeates every fibre of human beings. It is the precondition of existence, the product of chemical triggers and hormonal balances, a manifestation of personal identity and a powerful public and private symbol. Through sex we have opportunities to connect with other people, not just physically, but emotionally and from the deepest part of our being. Through sex we can also disconnect from other people, reducing them and ourselves to objects through which we hope to achieve solace, stimulus and the gratification of basic human needs and impulses. Whichever way it takes us, sex is a form of communication. Through it we are known. No wonder that it can excite public curiosity and evoke complex personal reactions.

This book considers sex in the context of adult couple relationships. It invites us to consider the nature of committed relationships and some of the life course issues that can affect the manner in which they develop. It offers ways of thinking about the problems that can surface in relationships between partners who know and are known by each other intimately, and some of the processes by which they may attempt to keep such knowledge at bay. And it considers the part sex plays in the theatre of close personal relationships. Taking a multi-discipline approach, the chapters provide important information about human sexual functioning, suggest approaches to helping couples with sexual problems and provide copious illustrations that bring it all to life.

It is common knowledge that sexual and relationship problems will present themselves more frequently to health practitioners than to specialists in the field, although often in disguised form. If those working with individuals and families, whether in health or other settings, are able to respond sensitively and appropriately to the often muted appeals for help in this area there are opportunities to make a substantial contribution to the well-being and development of sexual partners. There is a challenge for practitioners here. Working with couples requires competence in managing three-person situations, confidence in entering the privacy of the couple's 'bedroom' when invited to do so, and a capacity to judge when it is right to remain outside. Managing these boundaries requires a degree of self-knowledge as well as knowledge about other people. This book provides valuable information that will help readers think about what is involved, assess how far to go with couples presenting with sexual and relationship problems and equip them to make a sensitive referral if specialist help is needed.

Christopher Clulow PhD
Director, The Tavistock Marital Studies Institute
Therapies Editor, Sexual and Relationship Therapy
September 2003

About the author

Carol Martin-Sperry, an experienced counsellor and psychosexual therapist, has been working with couples for 18 years. She trained with Relate and London Marriage Guidance and manages a thriving private practice in London.

She currently runs a successful training course for counsellors, psychotherapists and related healthcare professionals who often have had little training in the vital subjects of relationship and sexual dynamics. Many of the concepts and frameworks in this book were originally developed for that training course.

She is on the team of BBC post-traumatic stress counsellors and has worked as a critical incident de-briefer, notably for the Ladbroke rail crash and after the 9/11 terrorist attacks.

Carol is a broadcaster, writer and consultant on counselling issues and represents the British Association for Counselling and Psychotherapy as a media spokesman.

She was educated at the Lycée Français de Londres and University College, University of London. She is bi-lingual in French and had an earlier career as a literary translator. She is married to Michael and has an adult daughter, Anna.

Acknowledgements

I would like to thank Phillip Hodson for pointing me in the right direction and encouraging me to start writing this book. Helen Perkes' extensive contributions have been invaluable throughout. I am very grateful to Dehra Mitchell for her helpful input and to Giuliana Orme for her support. Adrian Shire, Michael Maconochie and Anna Maconochie have been eternally patient in helping me with my minimal computer skills and Lily Morgan put the manuscript rapidly on-screen for me. Dick Blackwell's skilled supervision kept me on track. My experience with London Marriage Guidance was the original inspiration for this book. None of it would have happened without my editor, Maggie Pettifer, and her continuing encouragement, expertise and support. Thanks to you all.

Carol Martin-Sperry
September 2003

Introduction

All our clients are in a relationship, or have been or would like to be. And all our clients are living with issues about their sexuality, whether they are sexually active or not. Yet most psychotherapy and counselling training courses devote very little time and attention to these crucial aspects of our lives.

Freud, the founding father of psychoanalysis, was the first practitioner to talk openly with his patients about sex. Indeed, sexuality is at the very foundation of psychoanalysis. Yet as therapists and counsellors we collude with our clients in not mentioning sex, although it is invariably present in the room. This repression is a shared unconscious defence against anxiety because sex is such a personal, emotional and fundamental issue, particularly if absent. Ignoring it means excluding something very important and meaningful in the therapy.

In order to facilitate talking openly about sex, the therapist needs to make it feel safe. She therefore needs to be aware, informed and confident about the subject matter. The purpose of *Couples and Sex* is to bring a theoretical understanding of couples dynamics and psychosexual concepts to therapists who have already undertaken professional counselling or psychotherapy training to diploma level or higher.

Up to now, couples work in the UK has been mainly undertaken by Relate, who trains its counsellors to diploma level. Relate also runs psychosexual training courses and these are accredited. London Marriage Guidance runs similar courses.

The Tavistock Marital Studies Institute in London offers a psychoanalytic training in couples therapy. For psychosexual courses across the country, readers need to check with BASRT (British Association for Sexual and Relationship Therapy) who can provide information about current courses that meet accreditation requirements.

Because there is so little training available, one of the aims of *Couples and Sex* is to provide a theoretical and practical introduction. This book will therefore be of value to all therapists who work in private practice, healthcare, or other settings where people may present as individuals or as couples. There is a real possibility now that some general practices will encourage couples to be seen within the practice rather than be referred on to a separate service.

In such situations the therapist needs to look at each case individually and decide whether to refer on or work with the couple according to her expertise and experience. There is no doubt that those therapists for whom couples comprise the bulk of their work should be supervised by a therapist trained in couples work. The difficulty, though, is that there is a dearth of couples supervisors. *Couples and Sex* will be of value to supervisors who find themselves supervising couples work.

Three in the room is dramatically different from two. In couples therapy the relationship between the partners becomes the 'client' and the therapist is an unbiased witness who can be trusted not to judge or take sides. In addition to the basic skills of listening and reflection, and understanding and empathy, the therapist working with couples is also in the role of interpreter and negotiator.

There is often an assumption or expectation from clients that couples work is about rescuing the relationship at all costs. This is most definitely not what it is about. Like most therapy, couples and psychosexual work is about facilitating change or accepting the status quo when change is just too threatening. The outcome of therapy may be the end of the relationship and the mourning that comes with loss.

The relationship is the 'client' in couples work and its development reflects the psychological developmental stages of the individual. The relationship will have its conception, birth, infancy, its childhood, adolescence and maturity, its old age, sickness and death even. It will have a varying degree of ability to withstand internal and external events and crises.

Whatever one's theoretical approach, *Couples and Sex* aims to help one put the couple in a psychological, developmental and systemic context. When couples dynamics are fully understood one can also do effective couples work with an individual, if the client comes alone but with relationship issues.

Couples work requires belief in the unconscious and a basic knowledge of psychological development, as well as an ability to explore family patterns and to contextualise life crises and stages. The more cognitive and behavioural aspects include reframing of assumptions and expectations, problem solving, setting of goals and working with tasks.

Couples and Sex aims to give you skills and information that are accessible, practical and pragmatic. Much of the work is in the here and now, with an understanding of underlying causes, not just symptomatic effects. The book is divided into two parts:

Part 1 is all about couples dynamics.

Chapter 1 explains the theories about partner choice, psychological development and the Oedipus complex. It looks at gender roles and explains the use of genograms.

Chapter 2 describes the issues that need to be negotiated in every relationship, such as collusion, the balance between intimacy and autonomy, the expression of anger, and conflict and communication.

Chapter 3 puts the relationship in the context of the life cycle with its different stages and crises. It flags up the major flashpoints, such as having a baby, affairs, divorce, stepfamilies, and mid-life crises.

Chapter 4 is about process, and covers assessment and formulation as they apply to couples, and working with the transference and countertransference.

Part 2 is about psychosexual concepts.

Chapter 5 looks at the meaning of sex, psychosexual development, male and female genital anatomy, the phases of desire and what happens to the body during sex. It also discusses fantasy and masturbation.

Chapter 6 covers sexual abuse and how it affects relationships, paraphilias and sexual addiction. It describes the sexual assessment and genogram.

Chapter 7 is concerned with sexual dysfunctions and loss of desire. Remedial sensate focus exercises are described in detail.

The single hardest task in a committed relationship is accepting difference and the feelings it arouses. This includes difference in:

- gender
- race
- religion
- class

- culture
- age
- expectations
- family experience
- ways of communicating
- needs for intimacy and autonomy.

Working with couples is working with difference in the broadest sense.

Men and women are different. One has a thrusting penis, the other a containing vagina. The act of sexual intercourse is penetrative for men and receptive for women. Orgasm in men gets the sperm out; orgasm in women dips the cervix into the seminal fluid to help the sperm on its journey. The sperm penetrates the ovum; the ovum receives it. These are the biological facts and they have an important psychological resonance.

Our social development has been far more rapid than our evolutionary development. We are in danger of becoming out of touch with our primitive drives and instincts. Add to that the continuing confusion about gender roles, the cult of the individual, unrealistic expectations, an increasing desire for instant gratification and the accompanying low tolerance of ambivalence and frustration and it is no wonder that long-term committed relationships are becoming harder and harder to sustain in a social environment of rapid change.

The case material in *Couples and Sex* reflects the majority of relationships that present for couples therapy, and these are heterosexual. The theories and concepts apply equally to gay and cross-cultural relationships.

Throughout the case studies in this book, names and details have been changed substantially to preserve anonymity, but all cases focus on the common types of difficulties regularly encountered in couples work. For the sake of brevity counsellors and psychotherapists are referred to as 'therapists' throughout, and in all cases as 'she' – to avoid the repetitious use of she/he throughout the text.

Working psychosexually can be very directive and explicit, with a strong behavioural element. The therapist is often in the role of teacher and must be careful not to be perceived as abusive or exploitative. Boundaries and ethics must be rigorously observed. The therapist and the clients will be working in a very delicate, sensitive and personal area, often with material that may never have been talked about. The clients will have anxieties about the process being too invasive and revelatory. The therapist needs to be informed, confident and sensitive and able to share those qualities with the clients in a respectful way.

Psychoanalytic psychotherapy with couples used to take place with a male and a female therapist. This model is impractical in terms of resources, both financial and time-wise. The reality is that couples work takes place in many different settings, including GP surgeries, EAP companies (employee assistance programmes), voluntary and not-for-profit organisations, and private practice.

Therapists are often expected to know how to work with couples whether they have had any training or not, the assumption being that it is not that different from individual work. Therapists with no training in couples work are at risk of making clinical mistakes, getting pulled into triangular situations, being manipulated and generally feeling de-skilled. Talking about sexual problems is often avoided because the therapist is lacking in information and does not have the diagnostic or therapeutic skills that could help the clients.

While in no way replacing a full training, *Couples and Sex* will introduce the therapist to understanding and skills that will enrich her practice. It will give an increased awareness of the issues and processes that pertain to working with couples, both in the dynamics of what goes on between them and in the mechanics of their sexual relationship. The therapist will be able to make an informed decision about whether to take on a couple or refer them on.

PART 1

Couples

CHAPTER 1

Partner choice

■ Falling in love

Falling in love is such a powerful event because it puts us back in that state of newborn bliss. Our first experience of love is in that intense attachment to the mother who (ideally) gives us total care and attention, unconditional love and responds to all our needs. It is through this exclusive bond that the baby develops basic trust and security and the ability to be close and intimate in later life. Baby and mother are merged in a blissful union. But with love come separation, anxiety and the fear of loss and abandonment.

Falling in love brings the hope of reliving a union as perfect as the mother/baby relationship and the desire to be merged and never be alone. When lovers look into each other's eyes they are seeking the reflected loving gaze of their mothers' eyes, a world of safety and intimacy. But they are also connected to the fear of loss and the possibility of disappointment, frustration and anger.

The closer we are to our partners, the closer we are to our inner selves. Love can put us in touch with our inner strengths but it can also reveal the hidden feelings that have been repressed because they are unacceptable, shameful or too painful. We fall in love hoping to be freed from the problems caused by painful experiences. A profound relationship with the right partner provides a place of safety, an emotional container and a chance to work through past difficulties.

■ The power of romance

Romantic love as a basis for marriage is a twentieth-century phenomenon: the dream come true, the princess in the tower, the knight in shining armour, a fairy tale with a passionate embrace, a ride into the sunset and a happy-ever-after ending. This fantasy is constantly reinforced by the movie industry, by popular romantic fiction and by the media.

Marriage used to be a contract that brought two families together, with the dowry of property and land, goods and chattels. Being 'in love' was by the way. Today, at a time of rapid social change, the emphasis on the development of the individual – that is, personal fulfilment and the expectation of having one's own emotional, physical, psychological and sexual needs met – means that relationships do not always last for a lifetime.

With romantic love, if something does not work, there is often no attempt to put it right. The relationship is discarded in favour of a new one. People cut their losses and move on. The desire to keep feeling the thrill of the new means that we may ultimately be heading towards an age of serial monogamy.

Words used to describe the state of being in love include:

- ecstasy
- bliss
- passion
- thrill
- exciting
- intense
- overwhelming

- intoxicating
- blinding
- merging
- union
- wholeness
- yearning
- obsessive.

Is romantic love the right time to make a major lifetime decision about commitment to one person?

'We're in love, we have fun, the sex is great' is not enough. A marriage or long-term relationship is an activity for grown-ups who are prepared to share a psychological journey. It will reflect the developmental stage of each member of the couple. It offers reparation, an opportunity to put right what went wrong in the past.

■ Moving from 'in love' to 'loving'

A lasting relationship needs to transform from romantic love, which is both narcissistic and idealised, into something different. The couple need to move from fantasy to reality, from illusion to disillusion, from 'in love' to 'loving'. The relationship needs to be able to embrace the mundane and the ordinary. It is hard when the idealised love object falls off its pedestal.

So it is not 'I can't live without you' but 'I choose to live with you'; not 'I love you because you make me feel good' but 'I love you because of who you are'. It is not about getting one's needs gratified; it is about mutual caring and empathy. It is not about being merged, but about finding a balance between closeness and separation.

Couples set off on the journey with a light heart. Only later do they find that they have each brought along all their emotional baggage from the past. They fall in love with what they see in the shop window. Only later do they discover the hidden items and the mess under the counter.

Many couples are not bothering to get married. Yet the marriage vows are a powerful reminder that it is not just about the good times:

> I ... take thee ... to be my wedded wife, to have and to hold from this day forth, for better or for worse, for richer for poorer, in sickness and in health, to love and to cherish, till death do us part.

The yin/yang symbol, with its foundations in Chinese philosophy, expresses the idea of darkness and light equally held in balance in a containing circle with the seed of one contained in the other. Equally, this image can be applied to a relationship in harmony (*see* Figure 1.1).

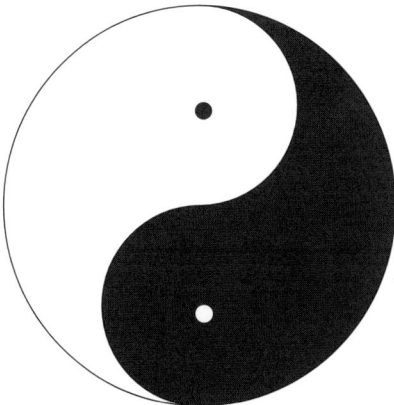

Figure 1.1 The yin/yang symbol.

■ Choosing a partner

Three factors make for a successful relationship:

1 Shared cultural and social values, such as ethnicity, social background, education, age group, religious beliefs.
2 Shared personal values, expectations, interests, habits, tastes and role behaviour with an ability to be tolerant, adaptive and co-operative, to accept difference and resolve conflict.
3 The capacity to meet each other's unconscious needs, to accept the unrevealed hidden part in each other as it unfolds or manifests, to cope with shared needs.

Similar family backgrounds and shared emotional functioning form a strong basis for a lasting relationship. A common experience of dealing with childhood difficulties is an important factor. Sometimes what a couple share is an inability to deal with emotional difficulties because they have avoided or repressed them and hidden them from themselves and others. What you see is not what you get.

Being in a successful relationship means not just accepting each other's blind spots but helping each other to see them.

When the psychological fit is right, each partner provides for the other the complementary bits in the emotional jigsaw that makes each feel whole. Therapy with couples helps them to identify the conscious and unconscious missing bits not just in themselves but also in each other (*see* Figure 1.2).

For example, when a shy introvert gets together with a gregarious extrovert, the hope (which may be unconscious) is that the extrovert will do the socialising for both of them and the introvert will be the quiet thoughtful one. Eventually, when it feels safe enough, the introvert will become a little more extrovert and vice versa.

The unspoken contract between the couple is that they can share their unconscious fears and fantasies. A good relationship with the right psychological partner gives them each a chance to work through past difficulties and to break repetitive patterns.

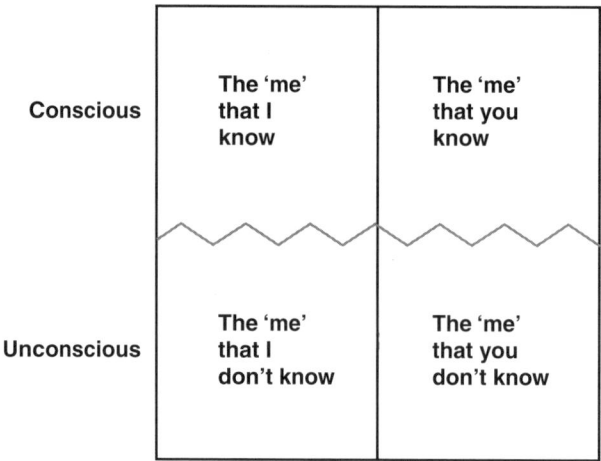

Figure 1.2 The psychological fit of couples: conscious and unconscious needs.

This depends, however, on how they have each experienced the developmental stages of childhood and growing up. These are as follows.

- *Birth to 18 months: ORAL.* This is when the baby learns about trust, intimacy, attachment, and dependence, through the experience of feeding.
- *18 months to 3: ANAL.* The issues here are autonomy, control, discipline and shame and are connected with the process of toilet training.
- *3 to 5: GENITAL.* The child discovers genitality in herself/himself and in her/his parents. The task is to work through the Oedipal phase, discover one's gender identity and deal with feelings of rivalry, jealousy and guilt.
- *5 to 12: LATENCY.* This is a time of learning and finding one's peer group.
- *12 to 20: ADOLESCENCE.* The issues here are of identity, sexuality, independence, separating from one's family, experimenting and rebelling.
- *20 to 40: ADULTHOOD.* The main tasks are to find a partner and a career path, bonding and intimacy, productivity and creativity.
- *40 to 70: MATURITY.* This should be a time of consolidation and fulfilment, with the ability to process personal and professional issues.
- *70 to ?: OLD AGE.* This phase is being redefined. The improvements in health and financial security bring a new energy and freedom. The final task is serenity, detachment and letting go.

Most of the problems of adulthood originate in difficulties experienced in the first three stages of development (oral, anal, genital), often with a replay in adolescence.

Marital fit and partner choice are about recognising in oneself and one's partner which developmental issues have been avoided or unresolved. The hope is of finding some healing in the strengths and experience of one's partner who has better negotiated those particular developmental stages.

It is also about expectations – couples need to ask each other the following questions.

- What do you expect of yourself in this relationship?

- What do you expect of your partner in this relationship?
- What are your expectations and beliefs about the nature of relationships?

■ The Oedipal story

The Oedipal story is at the foundation of Freud's thinking and therefore of psychoanalysis and developmental psychology. It is fundamental to understanding the dynamics between a couple and the origins of their difficulties. When a couple present for therapy one may be certain that unresolved Oedipal issues play a major role in their relationship difficulties.

At the heart of the Oedipal story is the incest taboo. The incest taboo is universal, present in all cultures and societies. It arouses primitive feelings and fantasies and strong defences. In Freud's developmental scheme the Oedipal phase comes after the oral and anal phases and corresponds with the ages of three to six years. The Oedipal phase is a time of psychological growth in the child, a time of conflict for the developing personality.

Around the age of three years the child becomes aware of genitality and engages in an unconscious and primitive struggle with each parent. This is a time of love and hate, of jealousy and rivalry, incestuous feelings and guilt, sexual fantasies and fears. The child is discovering her/his independence and is having to renegotiate her/his relationship with each parent. She/he is also becoming aware of the reality of parental intercourse and may have fearful and exciting fantasies about it. Her/his feelings will necessarily be conflicted and confused. The dynamic is repeated in adolescence with the added element of rebellion and sexual experimentation.

The Oedipal triangle is the original eternal triangle.

If the Oedipal phase is not negotiated successfully enough, unresolved issues may be played out later with the birth of a baby, where the father is in competition for love and attention from the mother (*see* Figure 1.3).

The eternal triangle may be repeated in an affair, with the same intense and conflicting feelings of love, hate, jealousy and rivalry, guilt and fear that were experienced in childhood.

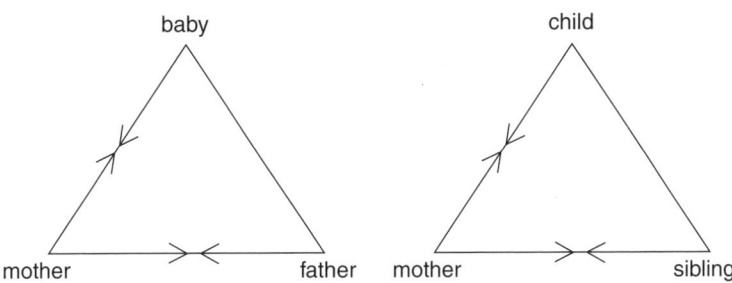

Figure 1.3 Oedipal triangles.

■ The myth

Oedipus is abandoned by his parents, Laius and Jocasta, king and queen of Thebes, because an oracle has foretold that he will kill his father and marry his mother. In order to prevent murder and incest, the baby is left on a hillside with a broken foot. He is rescued and adopted by the king and queen of Corinth and he grows up believing them to be his real parents. When Oedipus learns of the oracle's prediction, he leaves his home in Corinth to avoid committing the terrible crimes against his supposed parents. On the road to Thebes he gets into a quarrel with a stranger, who turns out to be Laius, and kills him. In Thebes he solves the riddle of the Sphinx and as a reward is offered the hand in marriage of the king's widow, Jocasta. Thus does Oedipus kill his father and marry his mother. When he discovers what he has done he blinds himself and is banished from the kingdom to wander as a vagabond.

During the Oedipal phase the child has strong feelings of love for one parent while having the other parent as a rival. The child's task is to give up the opposite-sex parent as an erotic partner and to identify with the same-sex parent as a gender role model.

If the parents have a satisfactory relationship the child is neither rejected by one parent nor seduced by the other. If the parental relationship is problematic the child may feel that her/his intense emotions are to blame. Jealousy of the parents' sexual relationship is a major feature. The child will literally get into the parents' bed to share the intimacy or physically separate them.

The mother/son bond can be very intense. A boy may actually say 'I want to marry you, Mummy' or 'Go away Daddy, I hate you'. His incestuous desire for his mother and his murderous feelings for his father can give rise to a lasting unconscious ambivalence and guilt.

Daughters also fall in love with their fathers but little girls do not have to separate from their mothers in order to acquire their identity. They do need to be empowered by their fathers in order to feel confident and special, particularly in adolescence when they become sexual. At that time fathers must maintain strong boundaries, without completely withdrawing, and mothers need to manage any competitive and rivalrous feelings while continuing to be a positive role model.

Unresolved Oedipal issues will surface again in adolescence when sexuality becomes conscious. Parents and children need to know how to handle intimacy, jealousy and rivalry. The shared task is achieving independence and separation so that the child can leave home and form her/his own relationships.

Example: **Mummy's boy**

Karen's marriage was in trouble. In a misguided attempt to improve the relationship, she decided to have a third child, John. John was very much the adored baby, but his father left when he was four. John only ever saw him very occasionally after that.

John and his mother had a very close relationship. His older sisters were young teenagers, so he grew up both spoilt and neglected, the way an only child often is.

His mother had a serious breakdown, triggered by the departure of her husband. At an unconscious level, John believed he had driven his father away, and made his mother ill. His guilt was such that he grew up feeling that he must never abandon her.

When her adolescent daughters left home, Karen grew increasingly dependent on John for emotional support and he became what amounted to a little husband. At the same time, as a single parent, Karen tried to be both mother and father to John.

Given his relationship with his mother, it came as no surprise that John's first relationship was with an older woman. It lasted for four years but ended because his partner could not cope with his mother's possessiveness and jealousy.

This was a pattern that continued to repeat itself in John's life. At first his mother's feelings about his girlfriends were not always overt, but before they knew what was happening, the partners were sucked into a powerful and destructive triangular set-up.

John never really grew up. At the age of 40 he was still at his mother's beck and call. His sisters had married and moved away. At some level John knew that he would not marry until his mother died. And by then it might be too late.

Example: **My heart belongs to daddy**

Vicky was the eldest of three children, the apple of her father's eye. She was a pretty, blonde, blue-eyed child who grew into an attractive and rebellious teenager.

Her father had brought her up to believe that she was special. His relationship with her was flirtatious but controlling. Vicky did not get on with her mother, who was plain and submissive. But, unconsciously, Vicky felt frustrated that, try as she might, she could not win her father away from her mother. She had lost the Oedipal battle in a way that was unsatisfactory to her.

At the age of 20 Vicky fell in love with an older, married man. She used seductive and manipulative behaviour to capture him. Part of the attraction was his initial unavailability and the illicit nature of the affair. Though eventually he got divorced and she married him, the marriage did not last long.

Vicky's second husband seemed more appropriate. But once he had fulfilled the basic function of providing her with a child, she grew bored with him. She started to treat him more like a brother and they got divorced.

Vicky gave up on marriages. She had a series of lovers who were all older men. One by one she discarded them when the romance wore off, as it inevitably did.

Throughout her relationships Vicky always turned to her father for help and advice. He remained the principal man in her life. He bailed her out in times of trouble. He wrote tough letters to her partners when (in her view) they misbehaved. He made all her major decisions for her.

But Vicky was barely aware of her father's power over her and seemed doomed to repeat her mistakes. Her partners could not compete and Vicky remained perched on the lonely pedestal her father had built for her.

The Oedipal story is present in every couple's relationship. Our first relationship with the opposite sex is with our own mother or father. That is the model we carry within us.

If that relationship has been a successful and fulfilling one we will look for a partner who is similar to our own opposite-sex parent in the hope of repeating that positive experience. However, if the opposite-sex parent has been idealised, no one else will ever measure up and we will always be disappointed. If the relationship has been difficult and problematic, we may feel attracted to someone very different. But because this is an unfamiliar experience we may instinctively want a partner who is similar to the opposite-sex parent, even if the relationship has been a negative one, because deep down that is what we recognise and know best.

The relationship with the same-sex parent is also very influential. That is the role model we identify with in early childhood. If it has been a satisfactory relationship, we are encouraged to be like that parent. If it has been a difficult relationship, we are determined to be different from that parent and not repeat their behavioural patterns.

So if a man has had a good relationship with his mother and has negotiated the right degree of separation he will be able to experience a similar degree of trust, intimacy and independence with his partner. If he has resolved any rivalrous issues with his father and identified with him as a man, he will be confident and self-assured as an adult.

Similarly, a woman who has experienced a positive relationship with her father will have good self-esteem and will be able to choose an appropriate partner. If her mother has been a good role model she will be at ease with herself as a grown woman.

A woman with a father who is weak and immature may choose a partner who is strong and firm in contrast to her inadequate father. But because this is unfamiliar to her she may find him controlling or over-responsive. A power struggle would ensue. Depending on how her mother resolved or failed to resolve any issues of power and control with her father, she may actively engage in it with her partner or opt out and give in.

Shakespeare has been called the first Freudian and the Oedipal drama is tragically played out in *Hamlet*. Hamlet's relationship with his mother Gertrude is a very close one. His father, whom he loved and admired, has been murdered by his uncle, who then marries Gertrude. Hamlet cannot decide whether or not to avenge his father by killing his uncle. How mad is he? Depressed, certainly, and unable to commit to Ophelia, who is tragically destroyed as a result of Hamlet's actions. Triangular relationships are a major feature (*see* Figure 1.4).

■ Diversity

According to the post-Freudian psychological developmental model the rationale for cross-cultural and multi-ethnic relationships can be found in the clients' Oedipal development. If the relationship with the opposite-sex parent has been difficult and unsatisfactory, she/he may unconsciously choose a partner of a different race or religion. This is an act of rebellion and rejection based on the hope that someone completely different will provide a completely different relationship.

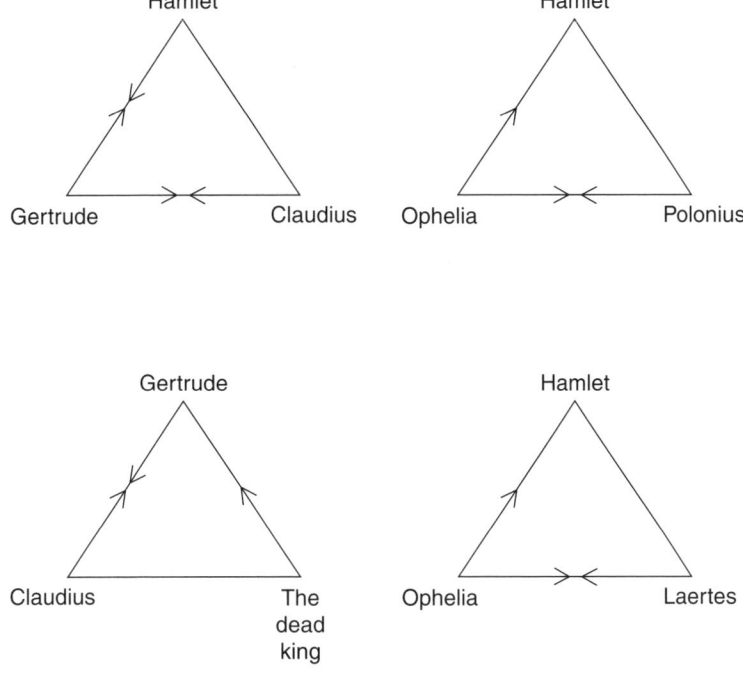

Figure 1.4   Triangular relationships in Shakespeare's *Hamlet*.

Example: **Caroline**

Caroline was the only child of an old-fashioned, authoritarian father and a submissive, downtrodden mother. Feelings were not shown in the family; everything had to look nice and normal. Her childhood seemed conventional and ordinary, but she felt the cold disapproval of her father and her mother's withdrawal.

By the time she reached adolescence she felt angry with her father for his rigid rules and with her mother for not standing up to him. Caroline chose to go to university as far away as possible from her home town, so as to get away from the stultifying atmosphere at home. There she discovered a world of freedom and tolerance, a heady mix of cultures and ideas. Caroline's boyfriend, Arthur, was black. The first time she took him home her father left the room when she introduced him. Caroline had triumphed, but her relationship with her father was permanently affected. Her mother was secretly pleased at her rebellious choice of partner, but it took a long time before she dared show it.

Meanwhile, Caroline was dealing with the difficulties of being a stranger in Arthur's family, who treated her with suspicion and contempt. It turned out that his mother also had a bold and rebellious nature, which is partly what attracted him to Caroline. When they left university, they lived together for a year, struggling with jobs and money. Caroline got pregnant. At first she was overjoyed. But she had a miscarriage and felt secretly relieved. She loved Arthur, but not enough to have his baby. The relationship came to an end, but not before they had shared a lot of soul searching. There was just too much difference to embrace, too many unrealistic fantasies and expectations about each other.

Couples in same-sex relationships may often have had problems with their parents that are rooted in their Oedipal development. If the same-sex parent has been cold and distant, or smothering and possessive, or controlling and powerful, she/he may look to the same-sex partner to make up for the love and attachment that has been missing.

Example: **Lucy**

Lucy grew up with a very strong father and a jealous, punishing mother. Her father taught her football and DIY but he bullied her. Her mother sneered at her for not being girly and feminine. Lucy was sexually abused by her uncle, but could not confide in her mother. She had a few unsatisfactory sexual encounters in adolescence but did not enjoy her experiences. Lucy gave up on men and remained celibate until she met Julie, who was a divorced single woman. Julie was warm and open and confident with her sexuality. Lucy found it comforting to be with her and gradually learned to trust her and be close and intimate with her. At first her sexual explorations with Julie were hesitant and shy, but eventually she was able to let go of her fears and bad memories and feel safe.

Coming out to her parents took a while. Her mother continued to put her down. Her father did not really understand. Lucy felt guilty and confused for a long time, which is what brought her into therapy.

■ The genogram

One way of helping couples acknowledge their areas of difference is to look at family patterns and attitudes, many of which are taken for granted. People get together with certain assumptions that they do not question until conflicts occur. These include:

- beliefs about gender roles
- how feelings are expressed, in particular intimacy and anger
- the value of money and success
- expectations of education and career
- messages about sex
- experience of illness, loss and death.

A very useful way of looking at family patterns is to draw a genogram. A genogram is a family tree that is also a psychological blueprint, a social and emotional
map. It includes births and deaths, marriages and divorces, and major life events
such as moves, schools, illness, previous relationships and affairs. It shows how
people in each family interrelate and interconnect and how certain roles and patterns of behaviour repeat themselves. A key to the symbols found in genograms
and an example to demonstrate their use are shown in Figures 1.5a and 1.5b.

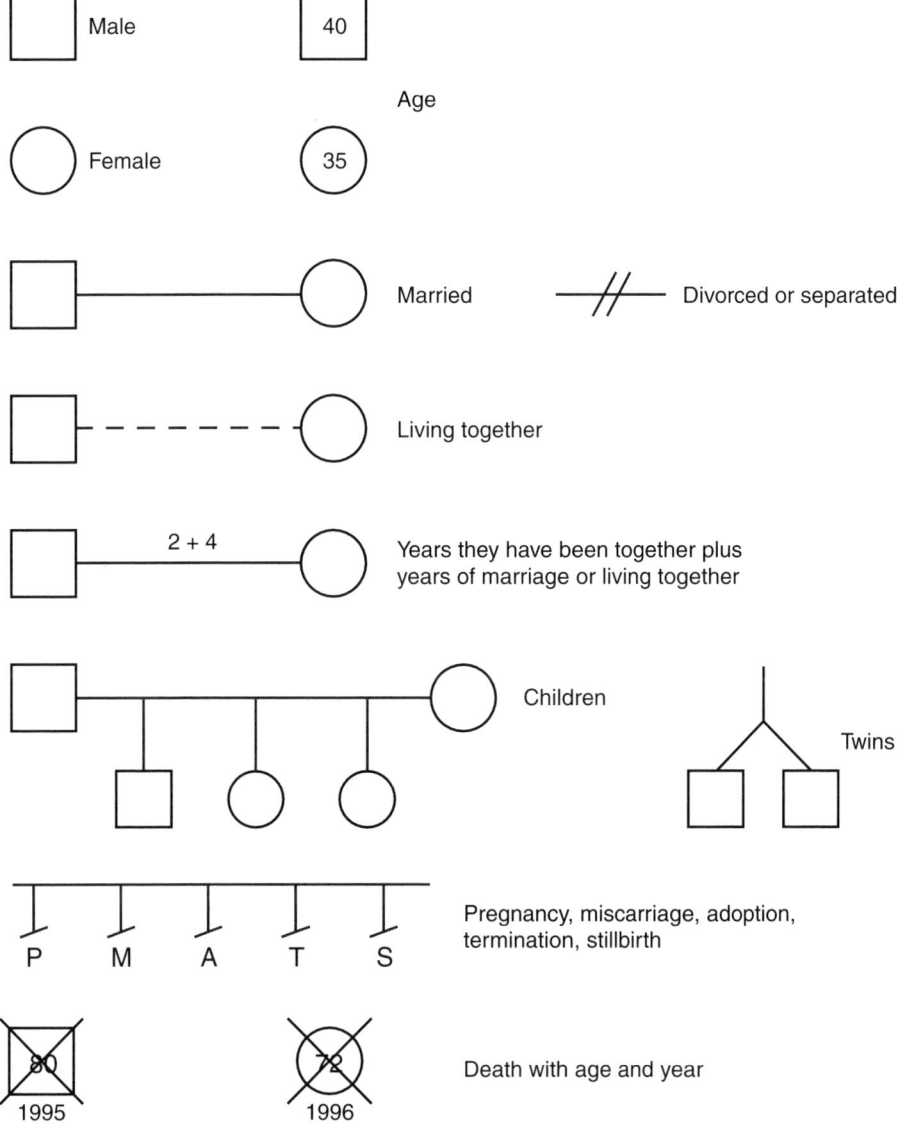

Figure 1.5a   Genogram symbol key.

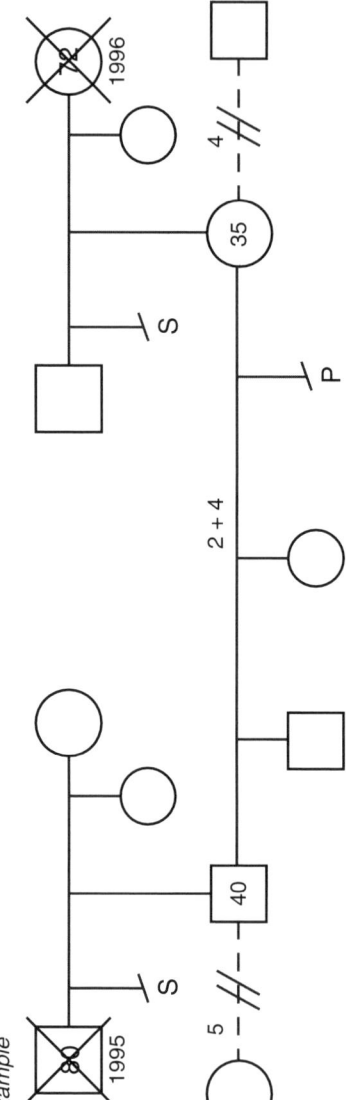

Figure 1.5b Genogram example.

Recognising these patterns brings the hope of changing them, of being able to do things differently. A genogram is not just about historical facts; it is a way of opening up memories and fantasies, secrets and family myths, and linking them to the present.

It is a fascinating source of information for the therapist and when shared with the clients it can be a powerful and instructive intervention.

If we look at the genogram of Diana, Princess of Wales, we can see repeating patterns and family events that explain why her marriage was never going to be an easy one. Figure 1.6 shows her genogram at the time of her death.

■ The genogram of Diana, Princess of Wales*

Much has been written about Diana's life and marriage. The circumstances of her birth may have led to her feeling unwanted from the start. She had two older sisters and an older brother who died at birth. As a replacement baby, she was apparently a disappointment. It was said that her parents had wanted a son, not another daughter.

Then came Charles Spencer, the much-loved son and heir. He shared with Diana the pain of their parents' bitter divorce and custody battles. She watched her mother leave the family home and was then sent straight away to boarding school at the age of six. She was not introduced to her stepfather until after he had married her mother. Her father married Raine when Diana was 16 and she was not told until after the event.

Diana first met Prince Charles at 16 when he was going out with her sister, Sarah, who was anorexic at the time. She described herself in contrast as 'fat, pudgy and unsmart'. However, her aristocratic family and conventional upbringing made her a suitable match. The Queen Mother and Diana's grandmother, Lady Fermoy, actively encouraged the relationship.

Diana's bulimia began during her engagement and lasted until after her divorce. It was probably a reaction to the panic she must have felt, and almost certainly a symptom of being let down and emotionally starved.

Diana had the ultimate fairy-tale princess wedding under the gaze of a world-wide television audience, a dream come true. Prince Charles needed a suitable wife, who would become the mother of his children. Diana was a lonely and neglected young girl from a broken family whom no one had paid much attention to. She was apparently insecure and needy with low self-esteem and a lack of confidence. Despite their backgrounds, she and Charles had contrasting personalities, little in common and no understanding of each other. They were also from different generations. Charles had little experience of intimacy in his family and did not know how to create it with his partner. He was an introvert who wanted as quiet a life as possible in the particular circumstances of his private life and the demands of his public role.

---

*The information presented in this account of Diana's life is drawn from a wide range of books and articles, all in the public domain, many of them based on the opinions of the author concerned. The synthesis of this information to illustrate the value of genograms in couples therapy is the author's own.

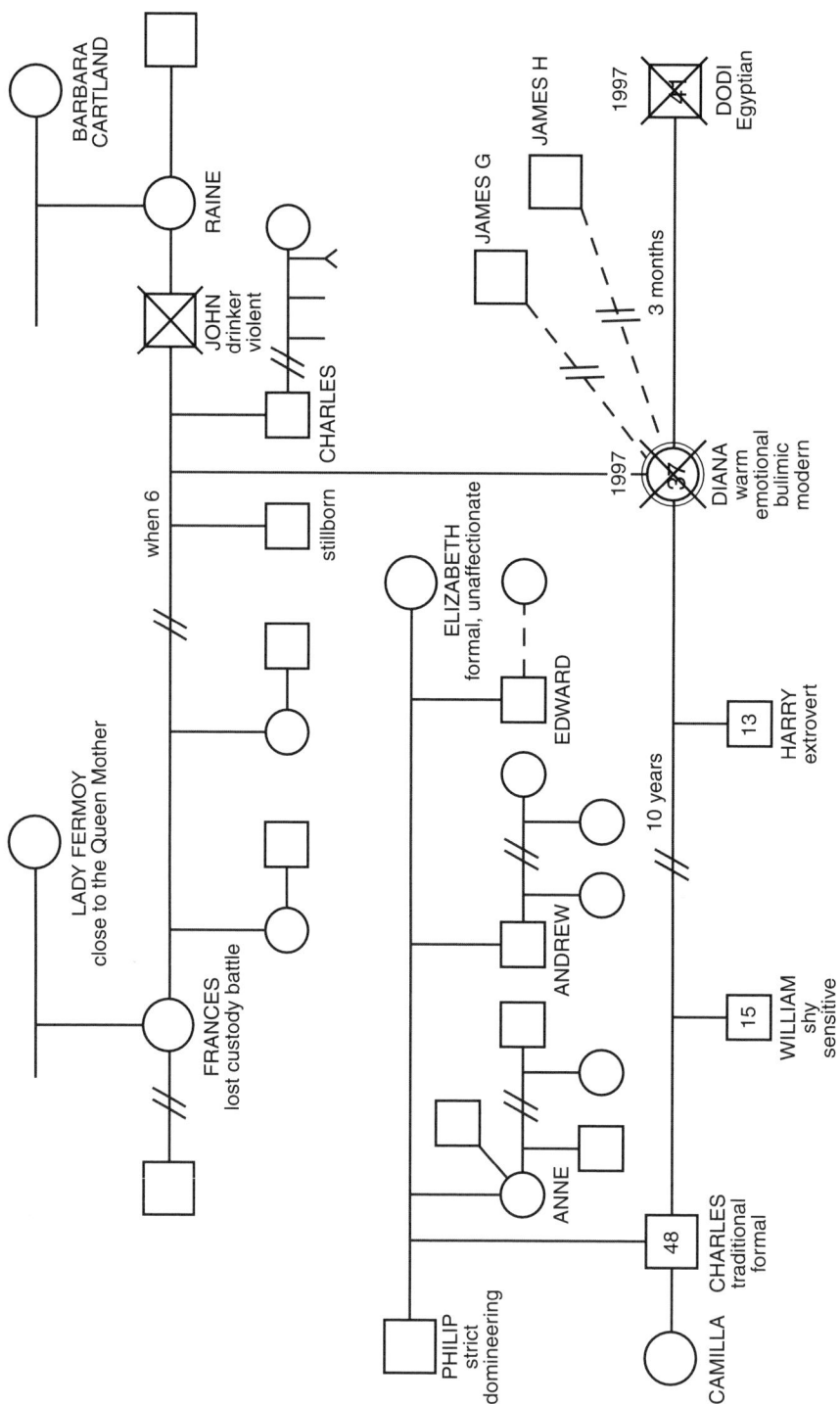

Figure 1.6 Genogram: Diana, Princess of Wales.

Diana was emotional, touchy-feely and spontaneous in contrast to Charles' formality and traditional reserve. She had a natural touch with people and was immensely popular from the start. The battle for media attention reached competitive pitch between them.

Prince Charles and his family were bewildered by Diana's mood swings and bulimia. Her behaviour became increasingly difficult – reputedly cutting herself, threatening suicide, and throwing herself down the stairs during her first pregnancy. She only succeeded in alienating her husband and his family, which in turn increased her sense of despair and isolation. They blamed the failure of the marriage on her bulimia and instability, but it was a vicious circle.

Diana was expected to cope with her role with little guidance or understanding from those around her. She was made to feel bad when she got it wrong and given little praise or encouragement when things went well. Her need for attention was played out in her complicated relationship with the press. She knew she could manipulate the media to her advantage. At the time of her death she was the most famous and glamorous woman in the world, a media megastar, a twentieth-century icon.

Prince Charles came from a stable and secure background and his position in the family as eldest son and heir to the kingdom was respected. His destiny was clear from the start and the rules of the game were formal and explicit. He grew up among loyal courtiers and members of the establishment in an atmosphere where duty and tradition reigned. However, he too suffered from a lack of warmth and intimacy within his own family.

Charles' parents were away for months at a time during his childhood. He was by all accounts a shy and gentle little boy who never gained his domineering father's approval and who was in awe of his mother. He was sent to boarding school at eight, followed by Australia, Cambridge and the Navy.

Prince Charles had several girlfriends, one of whom was Camilla. He felt he was too young to marry at 23, and while he was away serving in the Navy she married Andrew Parker-Bowles.

Diana was obsessively suspicious about Camilla's continuing role in her husband's life. She was accused of being paranoid but as it turned out she was right all along. Camilla would have been a far more suitable wife for Charles, with whom she had a lot in common.

Charles and Diana both came from dysfunctional families. There were difficulties in the marriage from early on. She was looking for an emotional rescuer. She needed a lot of affection, a secure and stable environment in which she could find some healing and be encouraged to grow and flourish.

She was the world's first post-modern celebrity princess. She wanted the freedom to express her feelings and put her natural sense of empathy and compassion to good use. This went against the grain of the royal family and the establishment who expected her to put tradition, duty and loyalty to her husband and the system first.

By the time Prince Harry was born Prince Charles was reunited with Camilla and the marriage was basically over.

Diana had two known affairs during her marriage, with James Gilbey (who nicknamed her Squidgy) and James Hewitt who betrayed her by writing a book about their relationship.

At the time Diana met Dodi Fayed in the summer of 1997 she was divorced and had matured into an independent woman. She was free from the oppressive atmosphere of the court. She had found solace in comforting the sick and the needy. She was a devoted mother who tried to keep her sons in touch with the real world.

Her complex relationship with the world's press led to her sudden death. The world grieved and mourned her with flowers and tears and a very personal funeral.

Prince Charles continued his relationship with the woman he had always loved.

■ Gender roles

The last 50 years have seen enormous changes in our society. These have been driven by economic, social and political factors that continue to develop and evolve at great speed.

Both men and women believe not only that they *can* have it all; they believe that they are *entitled* to have it all – a successful relationship, family, career and life-style. This raises important gender issues that affect relationships.

- Are gender roles interchangeable?
- Do men still see themselves as the main providers?
- How do women juggle their careers with raising a family and running the home?
- What is best for the children?
- Will the workplace continue to be dominated by competitive, aggressive 'male' values or will it become more flexible and adaptive, more 'feminine'?

Meanwhile, both men and women are turning into exhausted workaholics because their chosen lifestyles require keeping up the mortgage, going on foreign holidays, buying the new car, and paying for childcare. Where is their relationship in their list of priorities?

Men and women may have found real equality in many areas of their lives but biologically and psychologically men and women are different. Acknowledging and working with these differences is crucial to the well-being of the relationship.

Gender difference does not mean that men and women are opposed in some competitive power struggle or battle for control. Gender roles are complementary.

The most precious commodity in modern life is time. A useful way for couples to negotiate time is to ask them each to draw a pie chart showing how much time, in an ideal world, they would like to devote to:

- work
- family
- the relationship
- social life and leisure time
- personal time.

Then ask each of them to draw a pie chart showing how much time they actually devote to those five activities (*see* Figure 1.7).

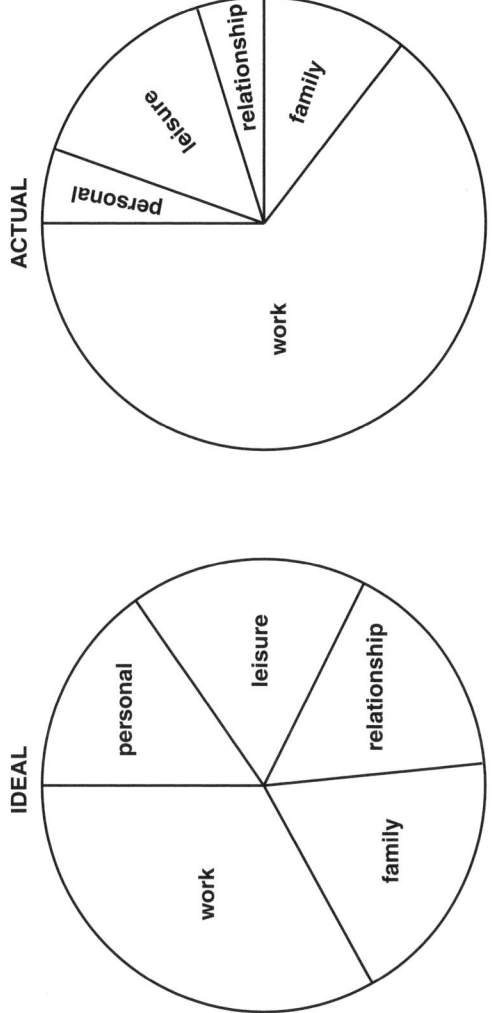

Figure 1.7 Pie charts: couples negotiating time.

These charts reveal a lot and provide many issues for discussion. Each person's priorities are highlighted, showing where the stresses lie, what sacrifices are being made and what expectations are not being met. Fundamental questions may be raised, such as how much do their material aspirations affect the quality of life? What price are they paying in order to have it all?

The post-feminist educated independent woman has increasingly taken on responsibility in all areas of shared life. New man is doing his bit in the home and with the children. But statistics show that up to three-quarters of household and childcare chores are done by the woman. Ultimately, women still tend to find their identity in their relationship, men in their work.

Freud asked the question, 'What do women want?'. Many are now asking, 'What do men want?'.

Are contemporary men feeling de-skilled, threatened and emasculated by strong, self-sufficient women? Is their self-worth and sexual power affected by the current status of women? Where does the modern woman fit into the traditional fantasy of mother/Madonna/whore?

It is a common male fantasy that the ideal partner will somehow combine the nurturing of a mother, the purity of a Madonna and the sexuality of a prostitute. When these roles become split in a man's fantasy, he cannot tolerate the opposing characteristics within the loved person, whom he experiences as a part object instead of a whole object.

The innocent girlfriend transforms into a sexual woman and then becomes a mother. Some men can no longer envisage the mother of their children as a sexual being.

A classic example of the mother/Madonna/whore split is Elvis Presley, who adored his mother and never recovered from her early death. Elvis met his wife, Priscilla, when she was 14. She became a mother at 23. It is said that Elvis never made love to her again after the birth of his daughter, and would never have sex with a woman who had had a baby. He did not remarry after his divorce from Priscilla and did not have any more children.

Many men unconsciously want their partners to care and look after them as well as their mothers did (or should have). And many women want men to be in charge and take responsibility so that they can be with their babies and little children.

Both men and women want a better quality of life. This may have to be negotiated with honesty in relation to each partner's true feelings, and not with a politically correct vision of how it all ought to be.

Example: 'Who does what?'

David and Jenny were a couple in their thirties with two small children. David ran his own business from home. Jenny was a successful solicitor. Both were achievers with high expectations. Jenny worked hard and was professionally ambitious. She was a strong, modern, independent young woman who demanded a lot of herself and of David. She had a younger sister with whom she had been in competition throughout her life for their father's love and attention. Her father, who was also a solicitor, was proud that she had chosen the same career as him and that she was so successful. Her mother, who was a quiet, browbeaten woman, did not understand her at all. Jenny did not want to be like her mother. (*See* Figure 1.8.)

David ran a landscape gardening business, which was affected by the economic climate. He was currently earning less than Jenny, but he was a hands-on parent. They felt they did not need a full-time nanny, but they did have an au pair. Their lives were very full, yet something was lacking. Their youngest child was nearly three and Jenny and David had not had sex since his birth. David felt rejected and unloved. Jenny was just too busy and too tired.

David was the youngest of four. He was close to his mother but he had seen what hard work it was for her to run the house and raise the children with no help from his father. His father was away a lot on business and his relationship with his children was somewhat cool and distant. David was determined not to repeat the traditional dynamic of his parents' marriage. Part of his attraction to Jenny was that she was so unlike his mother. But she seemed to have lost her energy and enthusiasm and, like his mother, complained of being tired all the time.

Jenny had been attracted to David's entrepreneurial spirit. She was ambitious, like her father. Yet after the children were born he had become more laid-back. Luckily she was earning a very good salary.

In therapy we explored their gender expectations. Consciously, they were meeting each other's needs for equality. But unconsciously things were very different.

Jenny did not want to be a traditional wife and mother, but she felt guilty and bereft at not being with her children. Sexually she had always been confident and assertive. She realised that secretly she wanted her partner to be sexually more dominant than her.

David admired Jenny's professional success, but admitted that he felt emasculated. He was also fed up with working at home, although he loved being with his children.

In the end they agreed that sacrifices had to be made in order to improve their relationship. Jenny agreed to take a year off; David took the risk of diversifying and moving his business to outside premises.

These changes took time and were quite daunting at first. Eventually they adjusted to their new roles and were able to renew their sexual relationship. Jenny realised that she had idealised her father and that David was not a replica. David knew that Jenny would never be a doormat like her mother and he would never be a distant father like his father. Both of them felt optimistic and empowered. They were relieved to have found a way of improving the meaning of their lives.

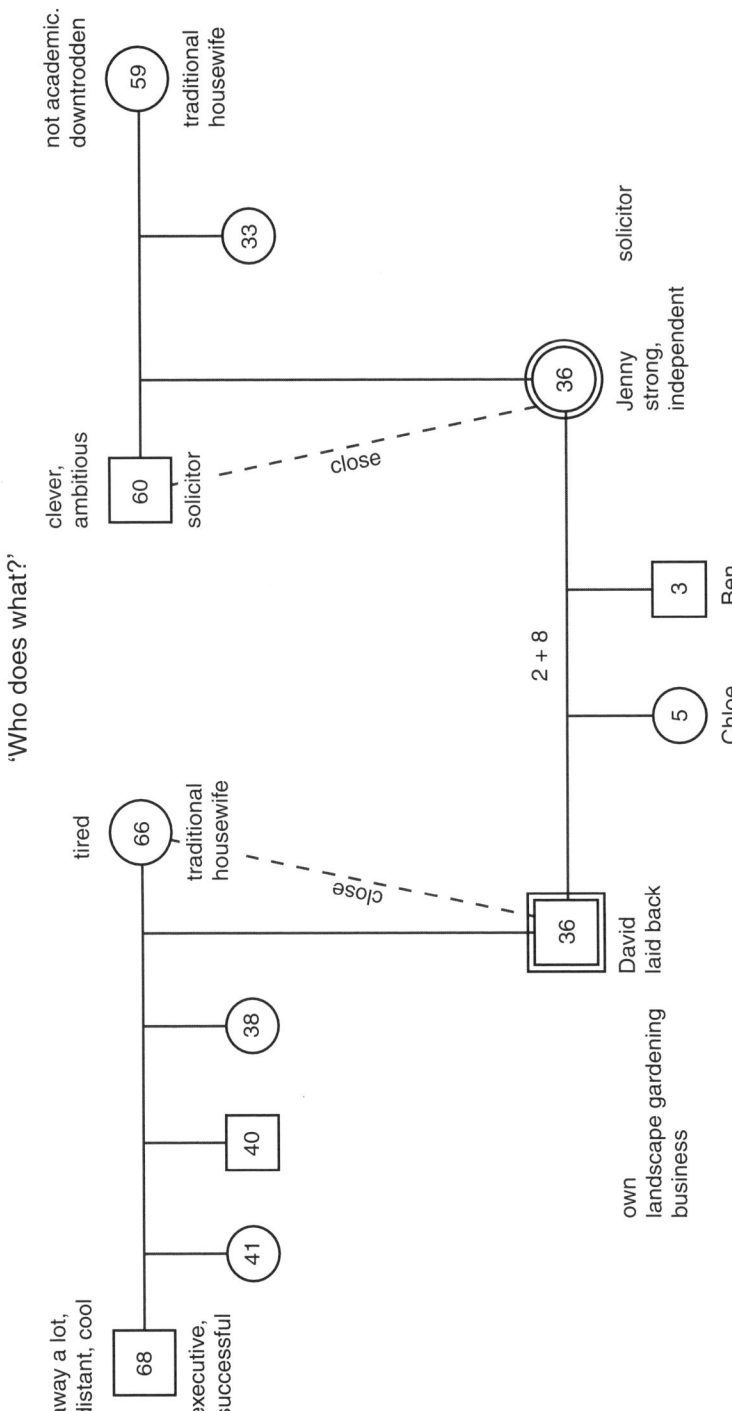

Figure 1.8 'Who does what?'

■ Unconscious forces and partner choice

The story of Sam and Ellen's relationship illustrates the unconscious forces that are at work in our choice of partner.

Example: **Sam and Ellen and the power of Oedipal triangles**

Sam was Italian, charming, social, extrovert. Ellen was Scottish, cool, mysterious, more reticent. He was 31. She was 35. They had been together for seven years. They had a four-year-old daughter. (*See* Figure 1.9.)

Sam was the youngest of four children. His parents split-up when he was six years old. His mother had two subsequent partners. He did not see his father again until he was 18. His mother was dominating and possessive, but much admired by him.

Ellen was the second of four children. Her parents had always put their marriage first, the children second. Her father was controlling, aggressive, frightening. Her mother put her husband's needs first and was submissive. Neither Sam nor Ellen had been given much physical affection in childhood.

They met and lived together in New York. When Ellen was seven months pregnant they married and moved to Milan. Sam was extremely unsupportive after the birth. Ellen was depressed and isolated. His father died at that time. She did not attend the funeral. They moved to London because she did not get on with his interfering mother. Sam and Ellen had very different expectations of marriage and parenthood, which reflected their childhood experiences.

Sam was the one who wanted sex. Ellen did not. He felt rejected; she felt criticised. He attacked her verbally; she withdrew. They were not able to function as a couple, or understand how the other was feeling.

Sam and Ellen had great difficulty in committing themselves to regular counselling and would often miss sessions or arrive late. This reflected their fear of commitment to the process and their difficulty in forming a trusting relationship with me.

It became clear from their family history that there were unresolved Oedipal issues on both sides. This was reflected in their interaction in the room. Sam would bully Ellen and boss her about in a controlling and authoritative way. She reacted as she did to her father – with fear and distrust.

Sam expressed a fear that she would find other men and always be withholding and ungiving with him, which is how he experienced his mother. This was reflected in his demands for sex and in Ellen's rejection of him.

I became aware quite early on of transference issues towards me as 'mother'. Sam and Ellen were competing for my attention and approval in the room, like jealous siblings. I was in danger of becoming the bossy interfering mother.

In the countertransference I felt a need to prove my competence. When I reflected this back to Ellen, we worked out that she had a fear of becoming a submissive wife like her mother. She also had fears about her own competence as a wife and mother.

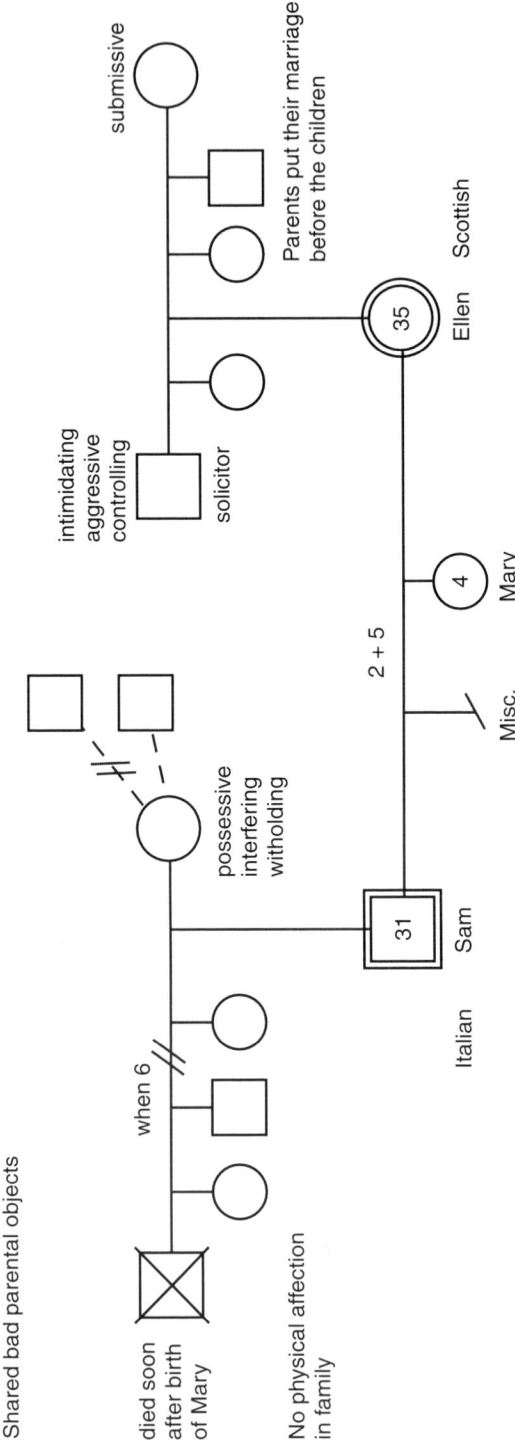

'Oedipal triangles'

- Different expectations of marriage and parenthood
- Oedipal issues
- His witholding mother, her aggressive father
- Shared bad parental objects

died soon
after birth
of Mary

when 6

No physical affection
in family

possessive
interfering
witholding

intimidating
aggressive
controlling

submissive

Parents put their marriage
before the children

solicitor

31   Sam

35

Italian   Sam

Misc.   Mary

2 + 5

4

Ellen   Scottish

His need for sex, her witholding

Figure 1.9 Sam and Ellen and the power of Oedipal triangles.

My interpretations helped put Sam in touch with his fear that if Ellen had too much autonomy and independence – that is, if she proved her competence, as his mother had – then he would have to leave Ellen just as his father had left his mother. Sam feared he would feel like his father: rejected and unloved.

Sam and Ellen's unconscious fantasies and fears of what it was to be a husband or wife were very different from their conscious expectations. Sam came to realise that he wanted a traditional wife who would run the house and be loving and giving. He imagined Ellen could fulfil that role. Ellen admitted to feeling ambivalent about the traditional role of wife and mother. She wanted a more equal relationship with more sharing of domestic responsibilities. Meanwhile, she had become defensive and unable to give affection.

They both had unrealistically high expectations of each other and they were projecting their need for a containing, good maternal object onto me. My wish was to be the perfect therapist as opposed to 'good enough'. Our shared task was to move from fantasy towards reality, to see if they could achieve a 'good enough' relationship.

It became clear that triangles were a major feature of the dynamic in this case (*see* Figure 1.10). We were able to look at several triangular relationships and their implications, for example:

- Sam, Ellen and their daughter
- Sam, Ellen and his mother
- Sam, his mother and her second and then third partner
- Sam and Ellen each with their own parents.

I was drawn into their power struggle as the third member of the triangle in the room. My part in it was both as the idealised good mother whose approval they competed for, and as the authoritative Oedipal parent who bullied them (his domineering mother, her aggressive father).

I was able to interpret these projections to the clients. Sam admitted how powerful his mother was and that he did not want Ellen to be like her. He also understood that his controlling aggressive behaviour frightened Ellen because it reminded her of her father.

They both acknowledged that they were deprived of parental attention in childhood. They understood that this made him needy and demanding but had made her punishing and withholding. The dynamic was acted out in their sexual relationship. We talked about this and they gained some insight into it.

They were now able to acknowledge the original marital fit. He thought she came from a traditional and united family and could replicate that for him. She thought he would liberate her from the tyranny of her family. In reality neither could give the other what he or she wanted or expected.

When Sam said he was ready to let go of his high expectations of the relationship, I felt that Ellen was winning the power struggle. She became more controlling, even castrating.

Just as I felt that we were moving into the next phase of therapy, they decided to stop coming. Sam had talked about separation, and had gone as far as finding somewhere else to live. But moving was too frightening – it represented a replay of his parents' marriage.

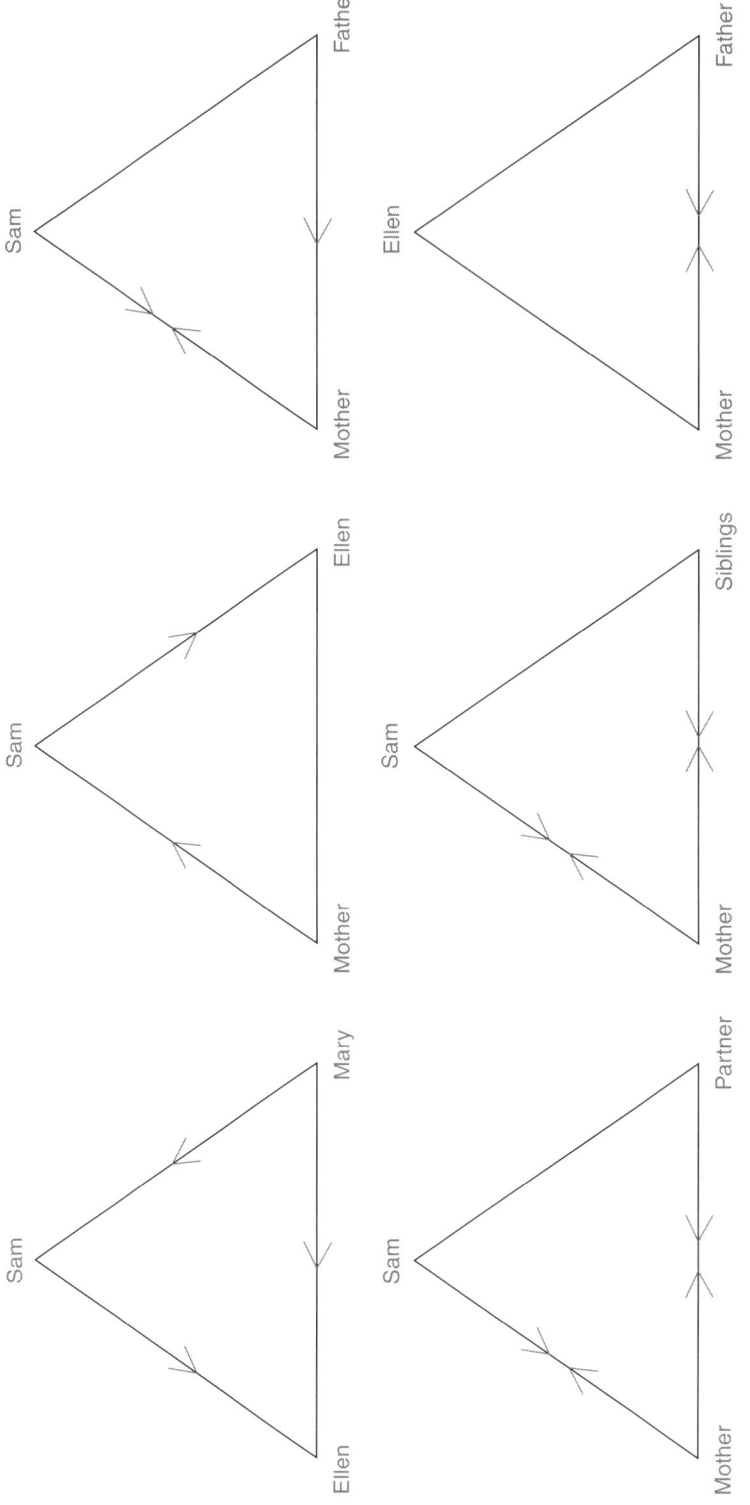

Figure 1.10 Triangular relationships for Sam and Ellen.

Getting deeper in touch with their unconscious material was also too threatening. They decided to stick with the status quo. In the countertransference I had also had an urge to end the therapy, because I felt they would not work as hard as I wanted them to – I was the authoritative, bullying Oedipal parent.

I understood that they had joined together in adolescent rebellion against me. Perhaps they needed to kill me off as an Oedipal object. In that way they could separate from their inner bad parental objects and start functioning as a couple.

This abrupt ending was a joint decision and proved that they could begin to take responsibility for themselves.

CHAPTER 2

Interdependence and co-dependence

■ Projective identification and collusion

One of the more difficult tasks in a relationship is keeping a balance between independence and dependence. Ideally, both partners should feel sufficiently connected to meet each other's needs without being overwhelmed.

The concept of projective identification is crucial to couples work. Projective identification is an interactive unconscious process shared by the couple, a mechanism for regulating unconscious feelings and fantasies.

When one has feelings that are unbearable because they are too painful or shameful, they get repressed. In relationships these difficult feelings can then be split off and projected onto one's partner who will carry those feelings on one's behalf.

This is an unconscious shared collusion. The partner's role is significant. The first partner takes on the projective identification because it also meets her/his unconscious needs. Because the other partner is now holding an important part of the first partner, the first partner has to control the other partner, usually with threats, promises, emotional blackmail and manipulative behaviour.

The partner's behaviour will be affected by the projections and she/he will act out accordingly. One can then blame the partner for her/his behaviour. The persecutory and destructive feelings of self-hatred and guilt can now be directed outwards onto the partner, who becomes hated and blamed.

This process enables one not to take responsibility for one's own feelings and behaviour while identifying with them unconsciously in one's partner.

The boundaries between the two partners become blurred; they are merged in a symbiotic tie. The relationship will feel uncontained, unsafe. But it serves a purpose because unconsciously the couple are sharing the same disturbing fears and defences (*see* Figure 2.1).

Example: if I am a very angry person who never allows myself to become angry, I may project the anger onto my partner, who will then find himself feeling unusually angry and behave accordingly. I can then criticise and attack my partner for his unacceptable behaviour while recognising and identifying with it at an unconscious level.

The major feelings in projective identification are:

- anger
- depression (*see* Figure 2.2)
- anxiety
- guilt

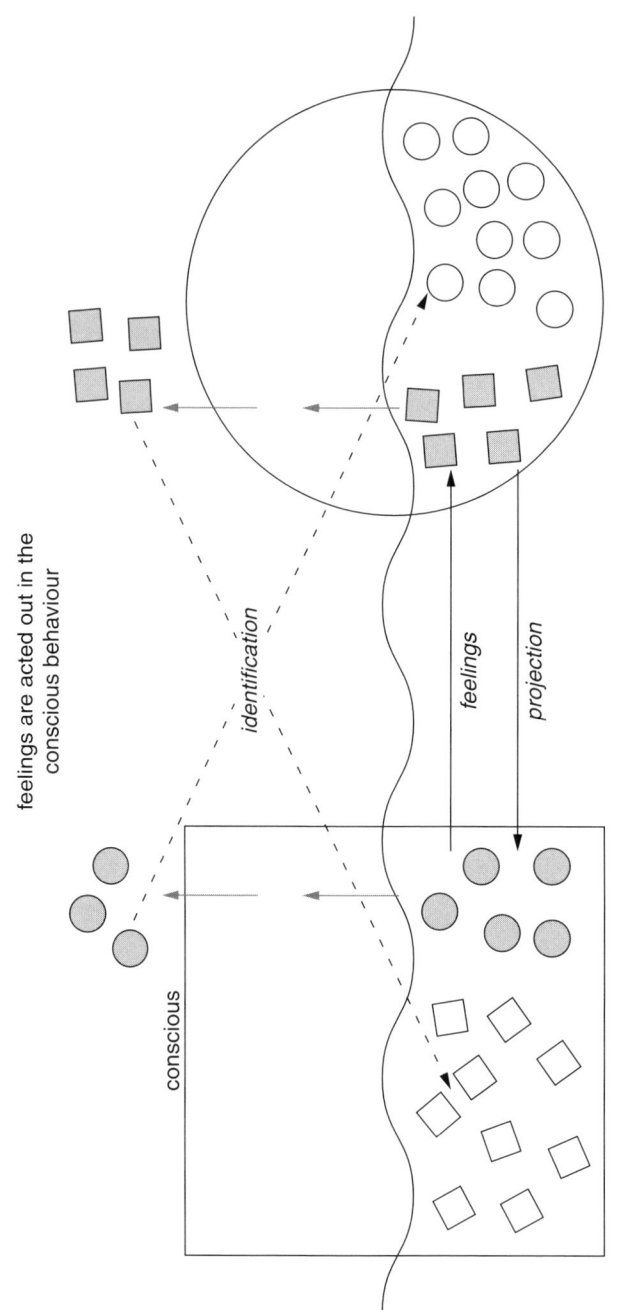

Figure 2.1 Projective identification.

- fear
- frustration
- hatred
- shame
- madness
- vulnerability
- helplessness
- hopelessness.

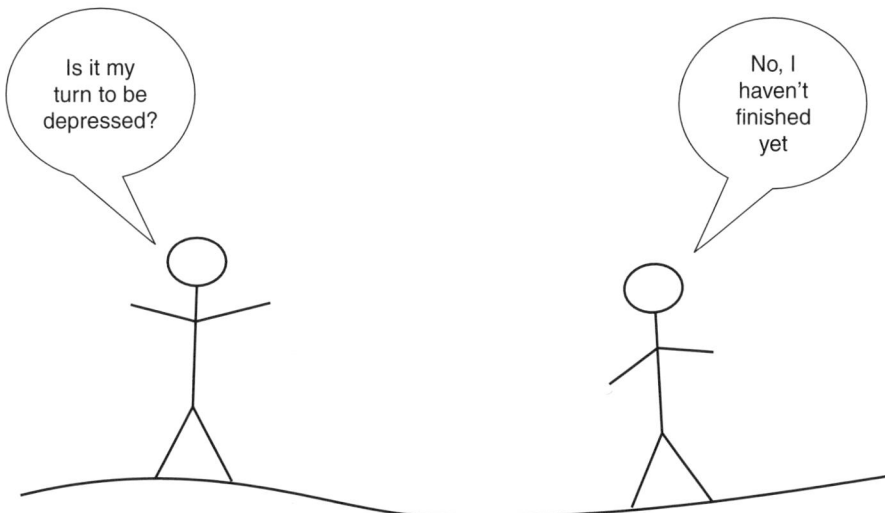

Figure 2.2 Projective identification of depression.

The projective identification may also be expressed in chronic or repetitive ill-nesses or psychosomatic symptoms such as:

- headaches and migraines
- backache
- irritable bowel syndrome
- digestive problems
- asthma
- eczema
- allergies
- sleep disturbance
- exhaustion
- myalgic encephalitis (ME)
- fibromyalgia
- auto-immune conditions
- gynaecological conditions
- loss of desire
- panic attacks
- phobias
- obsessive compulsive disorder.

Projective identification is a major factor in addictive/co-dependent relationships. The partner is controlled by the addict and adapts her/his behavior to fit in with what she/he believes the other wants, thereby giving up part of her/him self and losing an individual sense of identity.

Partners of addicts are often controller/rescuers. They hide the evidence, clear up the mess, pay the bills and look after the addict because it makes them feel useful and feeds their need to be needed. It also gives them a feeling of being in control of the situation. Sometimes they are martyr/victims, always seen to be doing the right thing despite the pain and suffering, in order to feel appreciated and get the gratitude they feel they deserve.

However, if the addict were to give up the addiction, the partner would have to take responsibility for her/his own behaviour, her/his own problems and unresolved conflicts. This is why the status quo suits the couple. They are operating in a closed system, in which change would be too threatening.

But who is the identified client and who has the problem? Clients will come to therapy and one will say, 'My partner has a drink problem. If only he'd stop, everything would be fine in this relationship', or 'My partner shoves and hits me, he's violent, I am innocent'. As always in couples work, one needs to look to the partner when one client is seen as having the problem.

Addiction can be defined as repeated and compulsive behaviour, which the person seems unable to stop, and includes:

- alcohol
- smoking
- illegal drugs
- prescribed drugs
- food
- gambling
- work
- sex
- love
- sport
- exercise

- violence
- self-harming
- drama
- adrenaline
- lying
- shopping
- computers
- TV
- therapy
- any other displacement activity.

The addictive activity may serve as an escape, an anaesthetic, a way of filling the black hole of emptiness and a way of keeping unbearable pain at bay.

Co-dependent relationships are those where there is a shared experience of damage, lack of self-worth, neediness and insecurity, of feeling not quite good enough and of pinning all one's hope of rescue, support and care onto one's partner. There is an unrealistic fantasy of being able to change the partner's behaviour.

These are often relationships where the partners cannot live with each other and cannot live without each other. The collusion lies in the unconscious agreement to share the same neurotic patterns and to buy into each other's behaviour because it meets one's needs.

Collusion confirms the false self in each other and gives it a resemblance of reality. It includes idealising the other as the holder of all that is good in order to make oneself feel good.

It is a joint defence mechanism against overwhelming feelings such as pain, fear, anxiety and guilt that originate in unresolved developmental issues and conflicts.

Each partner may have problems in the same or different developmental phase.

- *Oral collusion.* This is about sharing intimacy without being overtaken by one's narcissistic needs. How much do I give up to my partner; how much can I be myself? How much can I expect my partner to nurture me; how much does he expect me to look after him?
- *Anal collusion.* This involves issues around autonomy, power and control. Am I in charge in this relationship? How much autonomy can I allow my partner without feeling dependent and manipulated? Who has the power and control?
- *Oedipal collusion.* This is to do with aspects of sexuality and gender. As a woman, do I repress my inner masculine part for the sake of the relationship? Do I appear to be passive? As a man do I have to be strong all the time? Can I show any vulnerability and still remain potent?

How does the therapist work with projective identification and collusion in the couple? First, the dynamics and the patterns of behaviour need to be recognised and acknowledged. Then each partner needs to own what is theirs and hand back what is not. This requires courage, because the system at the very heart of the relationship is being challenged. It is likely that one partner will use denial, avoidance or a lack of co-operation as a defence mechanism. For example:

> *Partner A:* 'Yes, I may be angry, but I'm not that angry. Maybe you're *really* angry.'
> *Partner B:* 'But I don't get angry because it's too scary. It's better if you do it for me.'
> *Partner A:* 'Well, I'm not going to do it any more.'
> *Partner B:* 'But I need you to because otherwise I have to admit to my anger and deal with it. But I don't know how to and I don't want to.'
> *Partner A:* 'That's up to you. I'm not carrying your anger for you any longer. It doesn't belong to me. It makes me feel bad and act bad and then you blame and criticise me.'

Breaking the vicious circle of collusion and handing back projections enables the couple to demerge and find their own boundaries and the capacity to tolerate conflict, ambivalence and frustration in themselves and in the other.

■ Narcissus and Echo

Narcissus was a handsome young man who could not love or be loved and rejected the girls who fell for him. One of these was the nymph Echo. One day she followed him through the woods to a pool in a clearing. She had pined away so much for him that all that was left of her was her plaintive voice, which could only repeat what it heard. Narcissus saw his reflection in the pool and fell in love with it. When he said, 'You're so beautiful', Echo would say '… so beautiful', or if his words were 'I love you', she would say, '… love you'.

Narcissus leant forward to kiss the lips in the reflection, fell in and drowned. A white flower grew in that place, named Narcissus after him. Echo faded away.

■ St George, the dragon and the damsel in distress

This is another way of looking at the conscious and unconscious dynamics that occur between couples. The story seems so simple. The damsel (victim position) is being threatened by the dragon (persecutor position) until the knight in armour comes to save her (rescuer position) – *see* Figure 2.3.

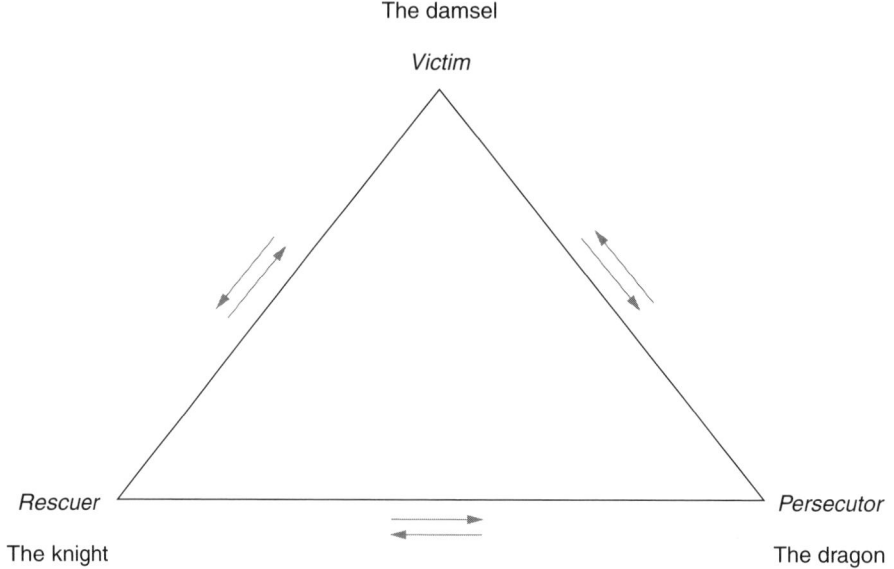

Figure 2.3 Victim/persecutor/rescuer triangle.

However, in relationships both partners can move from one position to the other, depending on the underlying feeling at the time – *see* Figure 2.4.

■ Projective and collusive couple types

- *Best of friends.* This is the contemporary model. Both partners are equal, sharing roles, responsibilities and tasks. The relationship is based on friendship and companionship. They are career focused and have no spare time, particularly for sex and intimacy, and can end up like flatmates or siblings.
- *Hunter-gatherer/nurturer.* This is the traditional partnership model. He goes out to work and earns the money; she brings up the children and provides a stable home. Gender roles are clearly defined. Their worlds are very different – workplace and home – so they often have limited shared experience and can grow apart.
- *Babes in the wood.* These are emotional orphans in need of rescue. Childhood difficulties have left them vulnerable and needy. They cling to each other in fear and despair, hoping that the other can be the adult in the relationship. They often have difficulties parenting.

Position	Attitude	Feelings	Behaviour
Rescuer	I'm OK. I help others. I know more than you. You are inadequate.	Concern and pity	Helpful
Persecutor	I'm OK. You're not OK. I'm better than you are. You're inferior.	Anger	Hurtful
Victim	I'm not OK. I'm helpless. You are better than I am.	Confusion	Helpless

Figure 2.4   Victim/persecutor/rescuer dynamics.

- *Fire and ice.* One is remote and unavailable; the other is emotional and warm. When frustration makes her hysterical, he backs off further and becomes controlling. She carries the anger; he represses his feelings. Because they are so different, they often feel misunderstood and rejected.
- *Cat and dog.* This couple thrive on constant fights and arguments. They blame and criticise each other continuously. The endless drama keeps the adrenaline flowing. Confrontation is a way of avoiding the real issues. They feel exhausted and demoralised, and isolated because they do not communicate effectively.
- *Victim/rescuer.* This relationship is based on a deal: 'I'll look after you because you are needy; you'll stay needy because I need someone to look after'. This is the dynamic of addicts, depressives and co-dependents. But if the weaker partner gets stronger, the stronger one becomes weaker.
- *Happily ever after.* This is the romantic couple who work hard to keep the honeymoon mood alive. The relationship is glamorised and idealised, and difficulties are glossed over. In a crisis it can all fall apart. The children often come second to the relationship.

Example: 'The caretaker and the wounded bird'

Sarah and Tom came to see me because she wanted more space and he wanted more intimacy. They were no longer communicating. She had been depressed more or less throughout the relationship. (*See* Figure 2.5.)

Sarah was a successful TV producer, aged 50. Tom was a partner in a consultancy business, aged 48. They had been together ten years.

Sarah had problems conceiving and had undergone fertility treatment early in the relationship. She had become pregnant but had miscarried. She had failed to conceive again. Two years ago Tom's business had moved out of London to Brighton and so had he. He did not like Sarah's London flat and she did not like sharing it with him.

They had both been married and divorced. Tom's ex-wife was a manic-depressive who had made several suicide attempts. Tom would not talk much about his family. He revealed that he had to be a good boy in order to get any attention or approval. Achievements were not celebrated. He was never praised or made to feel special. Anger was not expressed and was discouraged.

Sarah's mother was lively and intelligent. She had wanted a career and resented having children. She was frustrated and critical. Sarah felt disliked and disapproved of. She was never good enough. She could never get it right for her mother. In her mother's eyes her failed marriage and inability to have children outweighed her professional success. Her mother had given her a mixed message: be independent because men are useless, and find a man to look after you. Sarah was living this conflict with Tom.

There were two turning points in the relationship: the loss of the baby and the hope that she and Tom could be a family, and Tom's move to Brighton coupled with her refusal to leave London.

Because both Sarah and Tom had had previous therapy, they were quick to understand that their relationship was a very collusive one with a lot of projection.

Tom was a rescuer and caretaker. He was always very optimistic and smiling. Sarah was carrying his anger and depression as well as her own. Although she was ostensibly the independent one who wanted more space, she had projected her dependency needs onto Tom.

Her depression allowed Tom to care for her. This made him feel needed. He would not allow her to look after him. This made her feel guilty and depressed. Tom functioned better in the world by splitting off his negative parts and projecting them into Sarah. She unconsciously identified with them and acted them out. This made him feel better and her feel worse.

He was the sustainer of the relationship; she was the identified 'sick' one. If she did not need him to look after her, his fear was that she would leave and he would be abandoned and rejected. Thus he had an investment in keeping her depressed. His unconscious fear was that if he got in touch with his feelings of anger, fear and loss by letting down his defences and opening up, he would become the sick one. She would not be able to look after him and the relationship would fall to pieces.

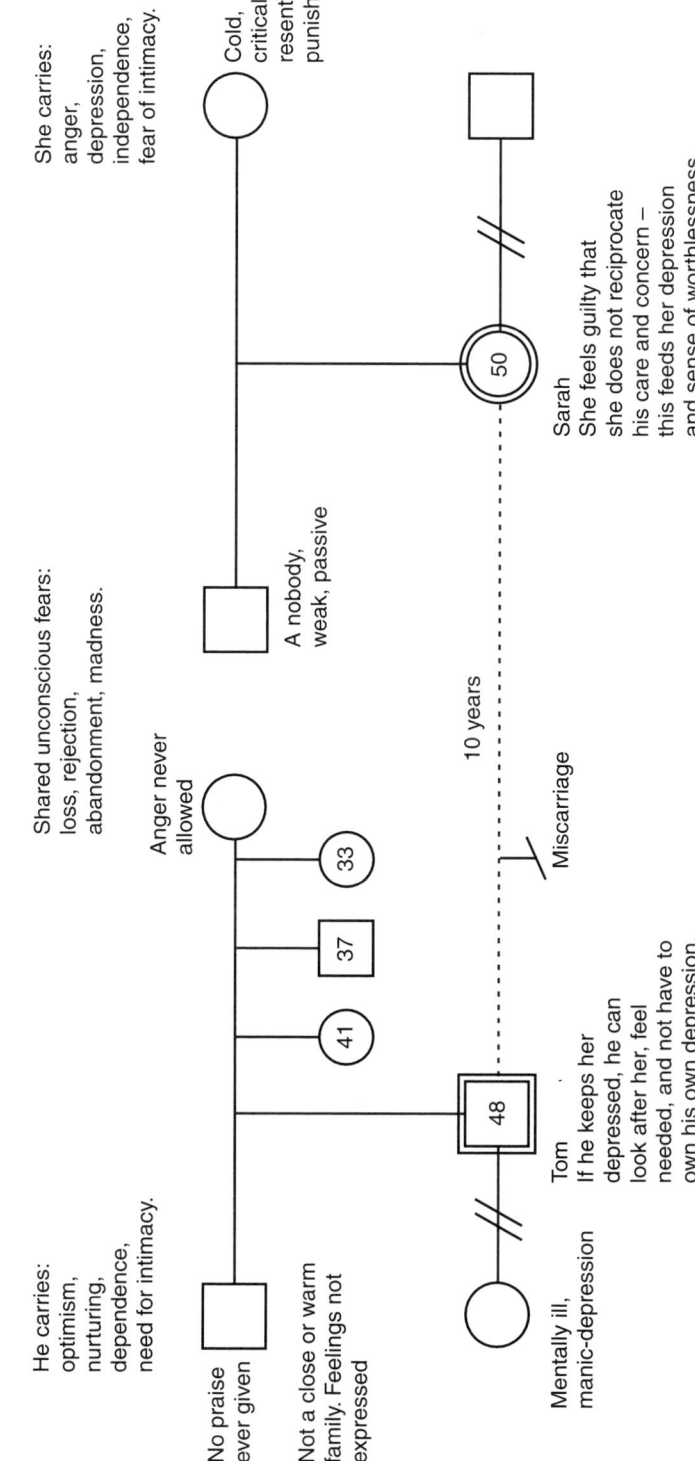

'The caretaker and the wounded bird'

He carries:
optimism,
nurturing,
dependence,
need for intimacy.

She carries:
anger,
depression,
independence,
fear of intimacy.

Shared unconscious fears:
loss, rejection,
abandonment, madness.

Cold,
critical,
resentful,
punishing

No praise
ever given

Not a close or warm
family. Feelings not
expressed

Anger never
allowed

A nobody,
weak, passive

Mentally ill,
manic-depression

Tom
If he keeps her
depressed, he can
look after her, feel
needed, and not have to
own his own depression.

10 years

Miscarriage

Sarah
She feels guilty that
she does not reciprocate
his care and concern –
this feeds her depression
and sense of worthlessness.

Figure 2.5 'The caretaker and the wounded bird.'

In the sessions Sarah complained that Tom did not express his feelings. But when he started to trust the counselling environment and his relationship with me enough to explore his feelings, she found it threatening. He closed up again and she accused him once more of not expressing his feelings. He colluded by encouraging her to talk about herself and her feelings.

These patterns of collusive vicious circles continued through several sessions. It was difficult breaking into the closed system they had created. Eventually Tom admitted that he could not allow himself to get angry, even though Sarah baited him in the session in order to get a reaction. He was afraid of 'going into meltdown'. When I challenged him, he would not get angry with me and made the connection with his mother: he was never allowed to be angry with her. And of course his ex-wife literally went mad when she was angry.

Sarah feared her anger was destructive and did not want to be identified with his ex-wife. So at an unconscious level they both curbed each other's anger and closed each other down emotionally. They had a shared fear of loss, rejection, abandonment and madness.

They both had a lot invested in the status quo. Tom was still very defended. Sarah continued to feel guilty and depressed. Yet Tom was now feeling safe enough to show some of his anger in the room. Sarah immediately attacked him and prevented him from further exploring these feelings during the session. Nevertheless, he was able to talk more openly about some of his fears and anxieties. Sarah again tried to divert the conversation and showed hostility towards me. Was she jealous of my role in the process of change? Was Tom now going to side with me against her?

Tom started using the sessions to reveal information about himself that he had not previously shared with Sarah. She was furious that he chose to do it in this way and with me. But gradually Sarah allowed herself to listen to Tom and to learn about his inner world. She began to acknowledge that he felt insecure and unloved. Still she did not know if she was able to look after him. Tom said he now felt resentful about her depression.

The relationship was beginning to change and shift around as they owned their projections and collusion, especially in the area of dependence and independence, anger and depression. Sarah then began to withdraw in the therapy. She was not sure if she wanted more change. Tom was now expressing fears of being sabotaging and destructive, some of which were projections from her. She was afraid of needing him. That felt too risky. He was now able to express his feelings. He was still concerned with rescuing her, but was far more aware of it.

As he grew more assertive, Sarah was perceiving him more as the critical parent than the enabling parent. In fact she had internalised a destructive critical parental object, a strong punishing super-ego. We spent some time exploring her difficult relationship with her mother.

When they ended the therapy, Sarah admitted that she found Tom's anger frightening, and hence to be discouraged. Tom owned some of his feelings of depression and worthlessness, which Sarah had been carrying. She still had difficulty in allowing herself to feel dependent and intimate but could talk about these issues more freely.

There was a strong sense of care and understanding between them. Despite their many unresolved problems, they were better able to share their feelings and make their unconscious fears and fantasies conscious. He still controlled the relationship with his thoughtfulness and consideration, she with her anger and depression. But they had much more insight and awareness.

I felt the therapy had ended prematurely. The splitting and projective identification were safely contained and explored. But they did not yet seem able to apply what they had learned in therapy to their lives outside. Change was still threatening.

■ Intimacy

Keeping a balance between one's needs for intimacy and autonomy is one of the hardest tasks in a relationship, particularly when the couple's needs are very different.

Intimacy is about sharing, trust, closeness, openness, honesty, warmth, empathy, connectedness, safety, harmony, privacy and uniqueness.

Autonomy means having a good sense of self, clear boundaries, a sense of existing as a whole and separate being, of feeling differentiated and contained while remaining connected to the outside world.

When the couple's needs are so different that they become polarised, splits like the following occur:

• intimacy	• autonomy
• closeness	• separateness
• togetherness	• space
• adaptability	• rigidity
• acceptance	• rejection
• enmeshment	• disengagement
• engulfment	• abandonment
• independence	• co-dependence.

True independence is tolerating closeness without it being overwhelming, and separateness without it being lost. One needs to have a good-enough sense of self and the ability to be alone in order to find the right balance between closeness and separateness in one's relationship. (See Figures 2.6a and 2.6b.)

Fear of abandonment brings the fear of loss of self. But fear of engulfment also brings the fear of loss of self. This is why the balance between autonomy and intimacy is so crucial and needs to be constant.

As ever, couples need to be able to understand and tolerate the difference in their needs and work through the issues when their needs become polarised.

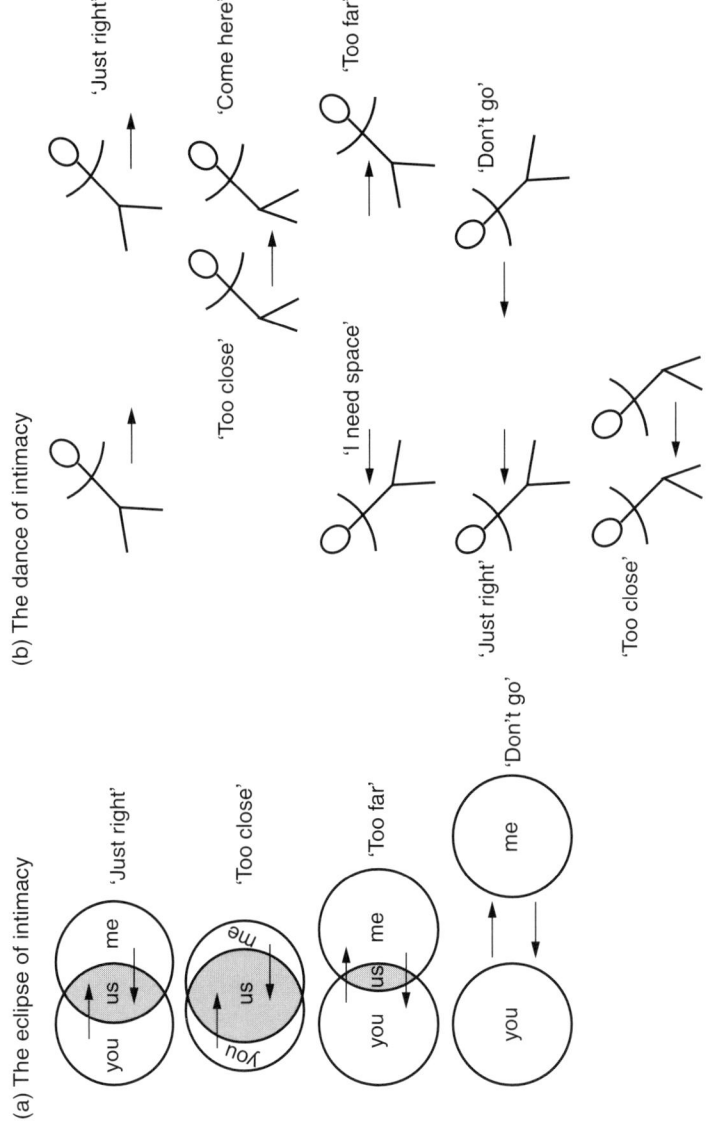

(a) The eclipse of intimacy

(b) The dance of intimacy

Figure 2.6 (a) The eclipse of intimacy; (b) The dance of intimacy.

■ Anger

One of the hardest emotions to handle in a relationship is anger. Expressing anger is often seen as threatening and destructive, yet repressed anger can turn inwards into depression. In showing anger people usually fall into two categories.

- *Volcano (hot):* a big eruption with sparks, steam and lava, which is usually over quite quickly and is followed by a dormant phase.
- *Earthquake (cold):* everything seems to be quiet, safe and reliable on the surface yet, underneath, invisible forces are at work. Without warning the earth will crack and split open. This is followed by the uncertainty of aftershocks before the earth settles again.

Anger can be experienced as overwhelming and frightening, or as something to dread. Volcanoes make a lot of noise and heat, but earthquakes mean one cannot ever trust the ground beneath one's feet. When a couple have difficulties with anger it is worth exploring the role of anger in their lives.

- How was anger handled in your family?
- Was it expressed or repressed?
- Did it lead to shouting and gesticulating, fights and violence, or days of silence and sulking?
- Was there one bad-tempered member in the family who did it on behalf of all the others?
- When you have an argument about something trivial, what are you really angry about?
- When you feel constantly angry with your partner, who are you really angry with?
- Who does your partner remind you of?
- Who are you really punishing?
- Are you aware of projecting your anger?
- Does your partner act out your anger on your behalf?

Anger carries a lot of destructive energy that can be turned inwards or outwards (*see* Figure 2.7).

Sometimes the energy is displaced sexual energy; sometimes couples need to have rows in order to feel passionate and aroused enough to have sex when they make up.

Anger can be addictive because of raised adrenaline levels or because of the calm that comes after the release of tension (like sex).

Anger is very often an unconscious expression of fear of intimacy, a way of sabotaging closeness. Then one can blame one's partner for the loss of intimacy (*see* Figure 2.8).

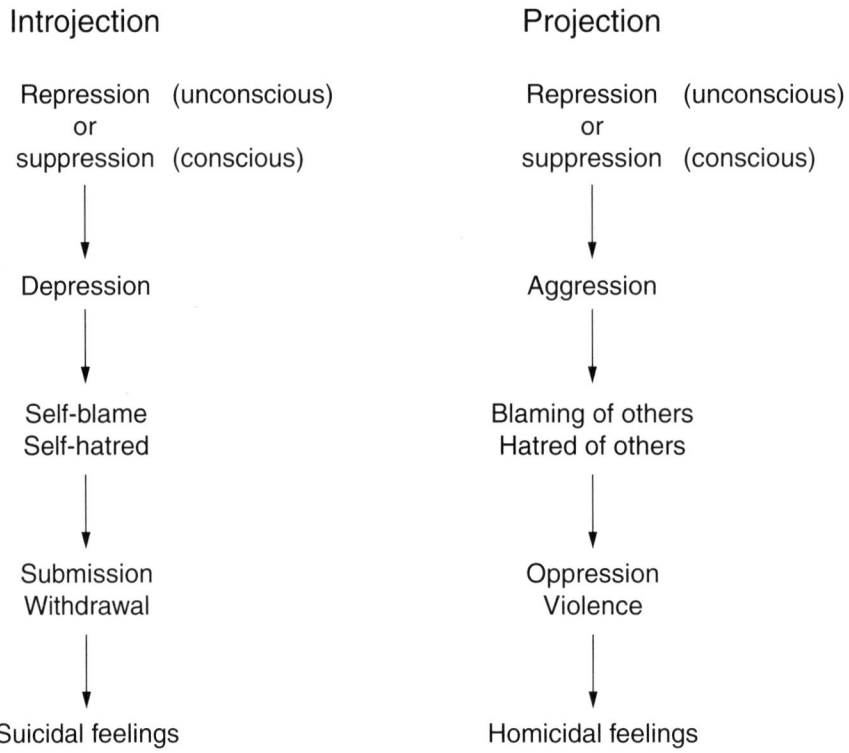

Figure 2.7 Anger: introjection and projection.

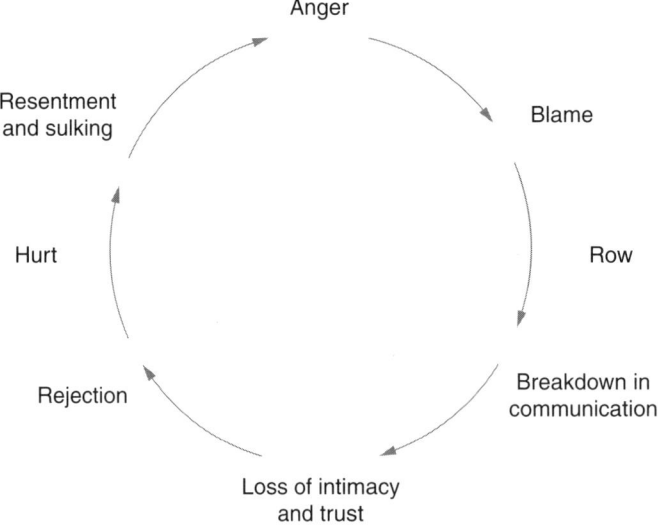

Figure 2.8 The vicious circle of anger.

■ Conflict and communication

Anger leads to arguments, rows, conflict and confrontation. Avoiding conflict is often seen as a major task in relationships, yet healthy conflict is an important part of any relationship. Couples need to trust each other enough to have a row and come through it. 'We never row' is not a good sign. Real connection means feeling safe enough in the relationship to express frustration, anger and annoyance.

When conflict is expressed in constant power struggles and battles for control, it is usually a sign of projective identification and collusion. The status quo suits the couple at an unconscious level. Change is too threatening to the system.

When couples are in the middle of a row, they are not in touch with their adult self. They are either behaving like competitive, point-scoring, manipulative children or like furious and demanding toddlers having a tantrum. Alternatively they may be in touch with the judgemental, critical, punishing inner parent (*see* Figure 2.9).

These concepts are readily understood by clients and are particularly useful to work with.

■ Good communication

The key to conflict resolution is good communication. If a couple can talk to each other, actively listen and be heard, then any issue in the relationship can be dealt with. This means talking without blame or criticism, listening without interruption, and reflecting back what one has heard.

Guidelines for good communication include:

- talking from 'I', 'me', not 'you'
- not making assumptions
- not speaking for one's partner
- not using 'should', 'could', 'ought', 'you always', 'you never'
- asking open-ended questions that do not require 'yes' or 'no' answers
- taking responsibility for one's own feelings
- sticking to the issue
- keeping to the present, not bringing up resentments from the past
- turning complaints and criticisms into requests
- checking out one's partner's expectations
- ensuring that one's own expectations are realistic
- being assertive, not aggressive
- not being defensive
- distinguishing feelings from judgements
- avoiding retaliation
- knowing when to apologise
- knowing what one realistically hopes to achieve
- giving to get
- making it a win-win situation, so there are no losers
- agreeing to disagree.

One of the hardest tasks in dealing with conflict is the ability to put oneself in the other person's place with genuine empathy. Both partners frequently have very

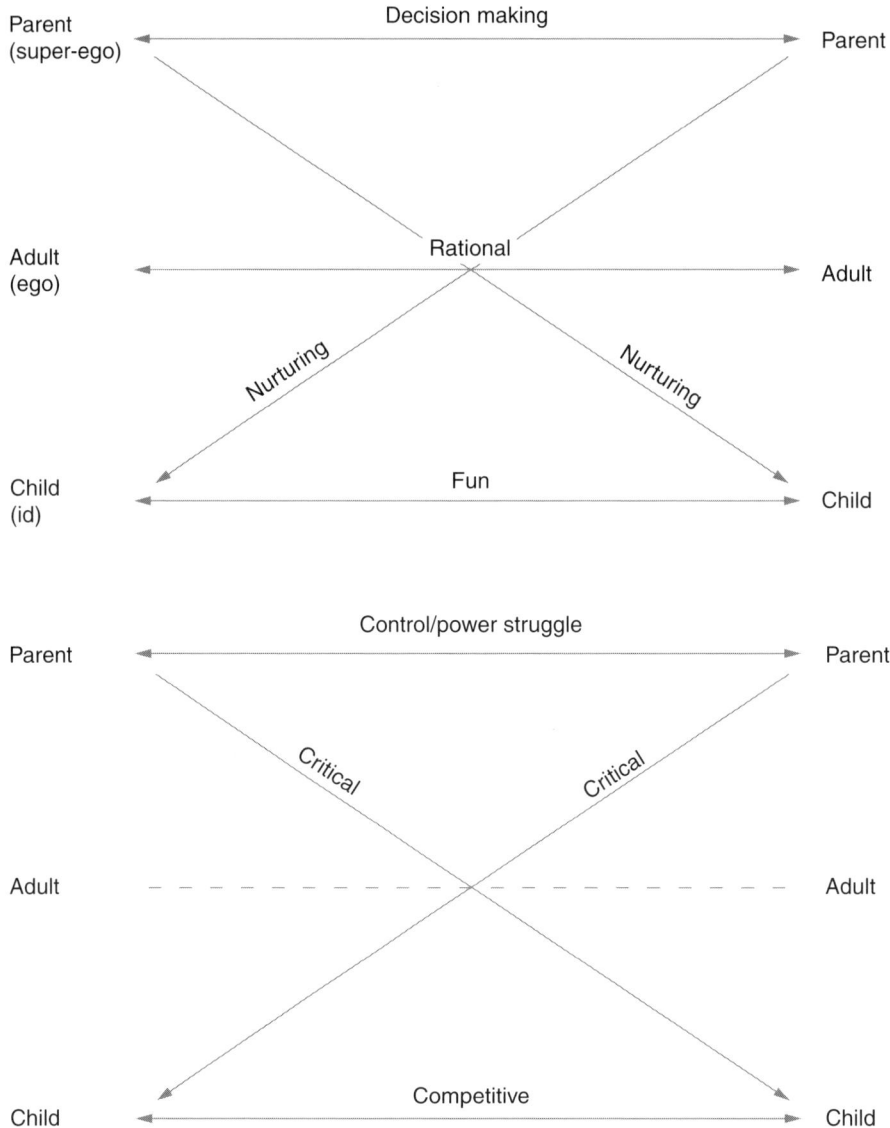

Figure 2.9 Parent/adult/child conflict and communication.

different perceptions of reality and events. They need to accept that both perceptions are valid, that sometimes there is no absolute truth, no right or wrong.

Gender differences also need to be acknowledged.

- Women tend to talk about their feelings.
- Men will usually try to solve the problem.

Although it is tempting for the therapist to act as negotiator, or referee, the most
useful way to help couples resolve conflict and communicate is to be a good
model in one's therapeutic technique (*see* Figure 2.10). The skills that are necessary

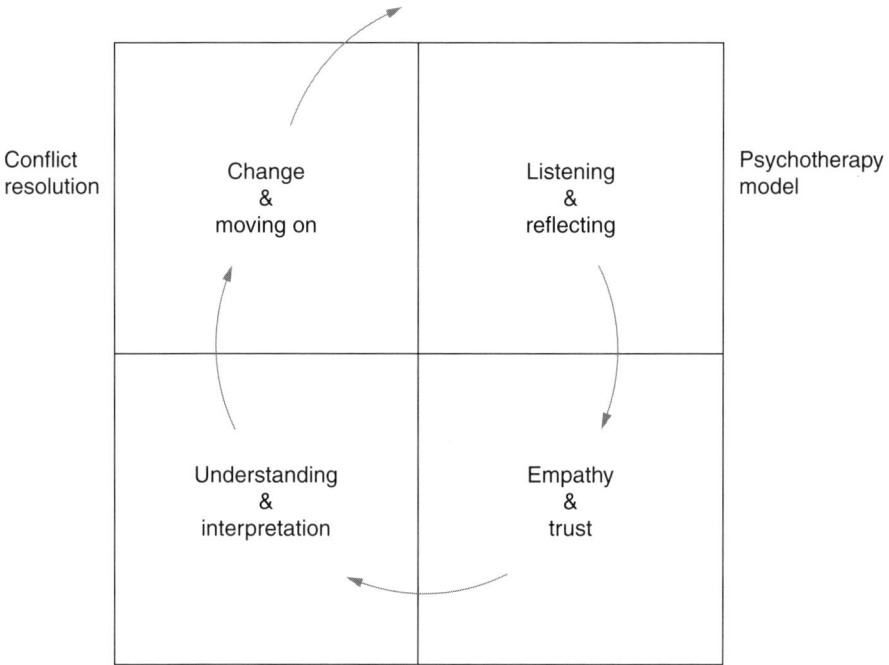

Figure 2.10 Conflict resolution: the psychotherapy model.

for good communication, negotiation and conflict resolution are the same as the basic skills of therapy:

- active listening and reflecting
- building empathy and trust
- understanding
- interpretation
- facilitating change
- moving on.

Communication exercises

1 Active listening
The partners take it in turns to:

- speak from the heart about feelings about the relationship, without blame or criticism, for an agreed length of time (for example, 5 to 10 minutes)
- listen without interruption to what the other partner is saying.

2 Looking
- The couple sit opposite each other and look at each other's faces in detail for one minute.
- They then close their eyes for one minute and recall the image of their partner's face.
- With that image in mind, each becomes aware of any thoughts and feelings, either positive or negative, and how it may be affecting them physically (heartbeat, tension, body language).

- They close their eyes for one more minute and see if this experience has reminded them of anyone else in their lives.
- They open their eyes and tell each other who else they see in each other and how that feels.
- They close their eyes again for one minute and become aware of what they were feeling and thinking as they were talking to each other.
- What would it be like to share those inner thoughts and feelings?
- How much do they feel able to share?
- Can they risk revealing their inner selves to each other?

3 Three instructions
The couple take it in turns to say the following to each other.

- Tell me something about me that you like.
- Tell me something that you think we agree on.
- Tell me something about yourself that you think I should know.

Repeat two more times.

When asking couples to do tasks it is essential to get feedback. The purpose of these exercises is to get the couple communicating at an equal level within safe boundaries. That way they can learn about themselves and their partners, share their feelings and feel confident enough to keep talking to each other.

■ Personality differences

Some of the issues that couples fight about are to do with their personalities. One can change one's attitude and behaviour, but usually one's basic personality does not change. Personality differences manifest in any of the following areas.

- Affection: touchy-feely   no touch.
- Feelings: expressed   not expressed.
- Needs: attention   admiration.
- Giving: generous   mean.
- Order: untidy   tidy.
- Money: spend it   save it.
- Language: Latin style (hot) Nordic style (cool).

When the couple are polarised in these areas and the splits become unbearable, it is time to help them ACT.

- **A**ccept difference.
- **C**ompromise wherever possible.
- **T**olerate what cannot be changed.

Sometimes one has to make ACT a FACT by adding:

- **F**orgiveness.

If you can't change it, don't fight it: go with it, embrace the pain.

CHAPTER 3

Life stages

Everyone experiences different events and crises in the course of their life cycle, many positive, some negative. Most crises come with change, loss, transitions and new beginnings. Couples may share a majority of these, but they may also be at different stages in their personal development and life cycles. This affects the development of the relationship.

When working with couples it is important to recognise the life stage of each individual as well as that of the relationship. The relationship needs to be seen in the context of the various crises and events that the couple have experienced and are experiencing. These include the following.

- Schooling – moving home – travel – adolescence – falling in love – sex – termination – accident – trauma – addiction.
- Living together/marriage – in-laws – miscarriage – infertility – pregnancy – childbirth – second baby.
- Affair – separation/divorce – new partner/remarriage – stepfamily.
- Career issues – financial issues – unemployment – redundancy.
- Mid-life crisis – menopause – empty nest – illness/death of a parent – grand-children – retirement – ageing – loss of health – bereavement – illness/death of partner.

A useful way to look at how the relationship is affected is to place it in the context of its own life cycle. The developmental stages of a relationship follow the same stages as the individual. Each stage brings up its own issues (*see* Figure 3.1).

- *Infancy (of the relationship)*: bonding, attachment, trust, intimacy.
- *Childhood*: fun, play, discovery, power-sharing.
- *Adolescence*: intensity, finding identity, adventure, experimentation.
- *Young adult*: taking on responsibility, commitment, autonomy, stability.
- *Mature adult*: productivity, fulfilment, power, experience.
- *Middle age*: change, transitions, new beginnings, re-negotiation.
- *Old age*: loss, resignation, acceptance, letting go.

There are, however, a number of possible flashpoints in the life of a relationship which need particular attention and awareness if the relationship is to transform and flourish. The rest of this chapter explores what those flashpoints are.

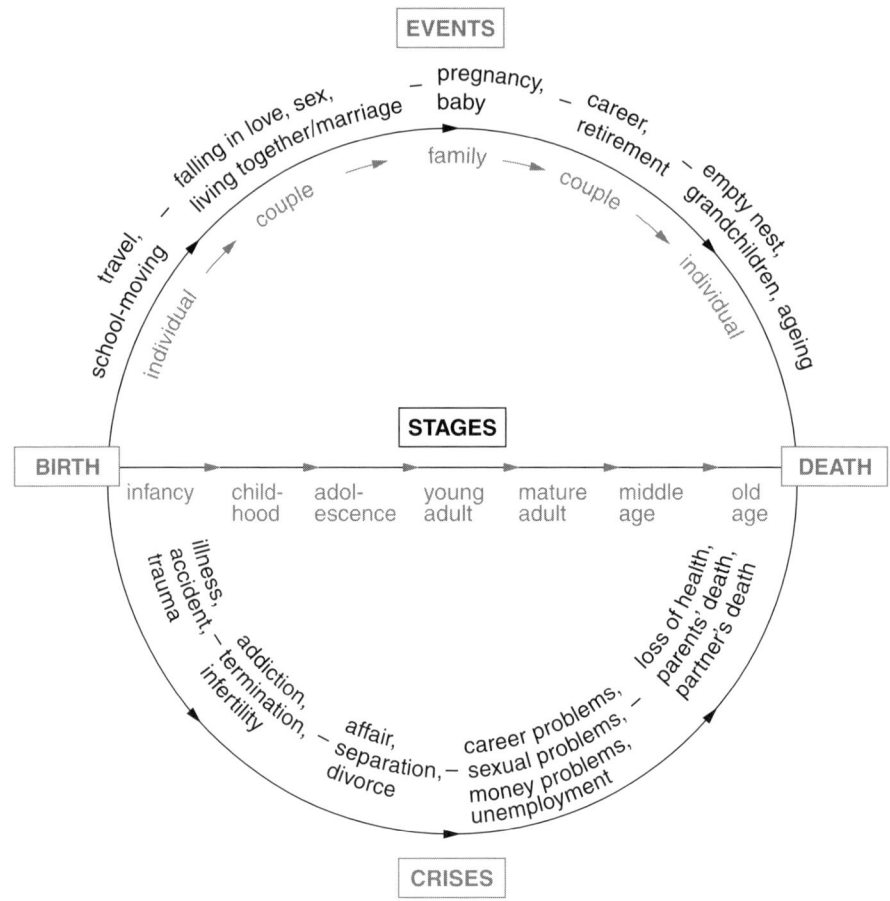

Figure 3.1   The life cycle.

■ Moving from 'in love' to 'loving'

This flashpoint may occur after several weeks, months or years of a relationship. Couples need to manage the transition from passionate romantic love to something less intense and more profound. There needs to be a shared ability to cope with ambivalence, accept difference and resolve conflict. The couple also need to be able to negotiate compromise and show tolerance for what cannot be changed.

Many couples break up at this point because of their high expectations and continuing need for excitement.

■ Having a baby

The birth of the first baby is the single most transforming event in the life of a relationship. It is the biggest irreversible change and a time of emotional upheaval and psychological readjustment. When a couple move from being two to being three, they need to understand that they will never be a couple alone together again until their youngest child has left home, by which time they will be at a very different stage in the life cycle.

Couples who are planning to have a baby need to do the things they want to do as a couple before having the baby. They may eventually split up as a couple, but they will be parents for life, and this will link them to each other beyond separation and divorce.

■ Conception

Changes to the relationship occur before pregnancy. If the decision to have a baby is a conscious and shared one, sex takes on a different meaning and becomes something very powerful.

If conception does not occur in the first few months, anticipation and hope are replaced by anxiety and disappointment. Ovulation kits appear. Sex has to happen at a certain and precise time and loses its spontaneity.

Treatment for infertility brings an increasing medicalisation of conception, with its cycles of hope and despair and the accompanying feelings of inadequacy and worthlessness, loss and bereavement, continuing uncertainty and failure. Sex is eventually replaced by test tubes and injections, blood tests and minor operations.

Pregnancy may occur only to be followed by miscarriage because implantation has failed to occur.

The effect of this process on the relationship is often devastating. The test of any relationship is how the couple manage crises together. Couples who cannot function as a team will revert to being lonely individuals and this will put their relationship at risk. The therapist needs to be particularly supportive and containing in these circumstances.

■ Pregnancy

Pregnancy experienced for the first time is an unknown territory. It can be a period of shared joy and intimacy but also a time of anxiety and questioning. During this lull before the storm there needs to be good communication between partners about their concerns and expectations. Some of the doubts and fears will be around the following issues.

- Will the baby be all right?
- Will they know how to look after her/him?
- Will they be able to give each other the support and understanding they will each need?
- Do they feel adult enough to cope with the responsibility?
- Will they feel trapped?

If the couple are in therapy during a pregnancy, this is not necessarily the time to do in-depth psychodynamic work, although some profound issues may well come to the surface. These need to be acknowledged, but the couple also need to be present in the here and now and aware of what is actually happening to them. There can sometimes be a shared denial of the situation. The couple carry on as though nothing has changed and are not really in touch with the process.

The couple's sexual relationship may be affected by pregnancy in different ways. Women often have an increased libido, or may not want sex at all, depending on how affected they are by their hormones and how they feel about their changing bodies. Men may find their partners particularly desirable and sexual, or they may not want any sexual contact at all. Anxieties about sex harming the baby are best addressed in the first instance with the GP or antenatal clinic. The therapist needs to help the couple to talk about their concerns and accommodate any differing feelings.

■ Childbirth

However well prepared the couple may think they are, no one can really explain the magnitude of this event, the shock to the system, the fact that life will never be the same again.

Couples often have unrealistic expectations of the process and feel disappointed when it does not turn out the way they had planned.

Most fathers want to witness the birth of their child and be supportive to their partners. Although they are not part of the physical process of pregnancy and childbirth, they can share some of the emotions. Some men do not want to be there. They are afraid of the blood and guts, of seeing the vagina in its functioning role, of witnessing such extreme pain. They may feel useless, guilty even. A few will be put off sex because they cannot bear to put their partner at risk of having to repeat the experience of childbirth.

Some women have many of the symptoms of post-traumatic stress after child-birth: confused feelings, hypersensitivity, fearfulness, raw emotions, helplessness. This is not the same as the 'baby blues', which typically occur on the fourth or fifth day, or post-natal depression, which may last for months.

No one can prepare a couple for the broken nights, non-stop feeding and chang-ing, lack of sleep and the ensuing exhaustion in the midst of emotional turmoil.

If she is breast-feeding, he may continue to feel excluded from the physical process. Furthermore her breasts, once his alone to touch and fondle, are no longer objects of desire. They are swollen, painful and functional, devoted solely to the needs of the intruder. Her intimacy and attachment are now primarily with the baby.

While she needs support, encouragement and reassurance, who is going to give that to him? He is no longer her number one priority, the centre of attention. He has been displaced. Some men find it hard to bear and escape into work or have an affair.

Meanwhile she is dealing with at least a year of surplus hormones and a body that will never quite be the same again. Whose body is it? Hers, his or the baby's? Mother, partner, worker? Many women lose their sense of identity and sense of self. They no longer know what their role is. Huge demands are being made on them. The freedom and independence they took for granted are replaced by major responsibility and a feeling of being trapped.

- How can they find time and energy for their relationship? With great difficulty. Will they ever have sex again? Yes, but not for a while, or for a long while in some cases.

- Couples in therapy at this stage of their lives will have some issues about their families of origin, their experiences of their own childhood and the parenting they received. They will come with assumptions, expectations and hopes that they may not have shared with each other. This is a chance for them to make it different for their own child, not to repeat their parents' behaviour, and to find some healing of their own childhood wounds.
- New parents often feel resentful about the baby, angry and hateful even, but are too guilty to share those feelings with each other.
- Their sexual relationship may need rebuilding. She now knows that sex has consequences. He may now see her as a mother and not a sexual being. There could be major adjustments to be made.

Couples may each have different ideas about how to bring up their child, which could lead to long-term arguments and power struggles. They need to know how to resolve their differences, function together as a team and act consistently as parents. With less support from families and the community, therapy will be a safe place for them to communicate and explore their feelings. The therapist will be experienced as a transferential good mother.

The positive side of parenthood for a couple is shared love, pride, fulfilment and commitment. It will bring meaning and purpose to their lives, a sense of intense happiness and joy and an increasingly profound bond. This too can be acknowledged in therapy, if they have not found a way of expressing it to each other.

If the couple have managed the transition to parenthood in a 'good-enough' way, it will feel safe for them to have a second baby. However, some couples fall apart after the second baby. Men often feel even more trapped than after the first birth. Their relationship has been taken over by domesticity and family issues. If they are experiencing unresolved Oedipal issues of jealousy and rivalry they may start a new relationship.

Some women feel so empowered by their children that they no longer need their partners. They have got their babies, they do not want sex any more, they can provide for themselves. What is the man for?

In both cases the abandoned partner will feel rejected and betrayed and will need therapeutic support.

Example: **'And baby makes three'** (*see* **Figure 3.2**)

Freddie and Alison had not had sex since the birth of their son Luke, now two. Freddie felt jealous and resentful; she felt he was not there for her. They had frequent rows, which were destructive and abusive. There was neither trust nor intimacy between them.

They said they wanted to accept their differences, care for each other and resume their sexual relationship.

Alison, 30, was a shop assistant. She came from a large family that was ruled by a manipulative mother who shouted and hit her children. She felt emotionally abused and a victim of her parents' volatile relationship. She also felt incapable of being in a trusting and loving relationship, because she had little experience of one.

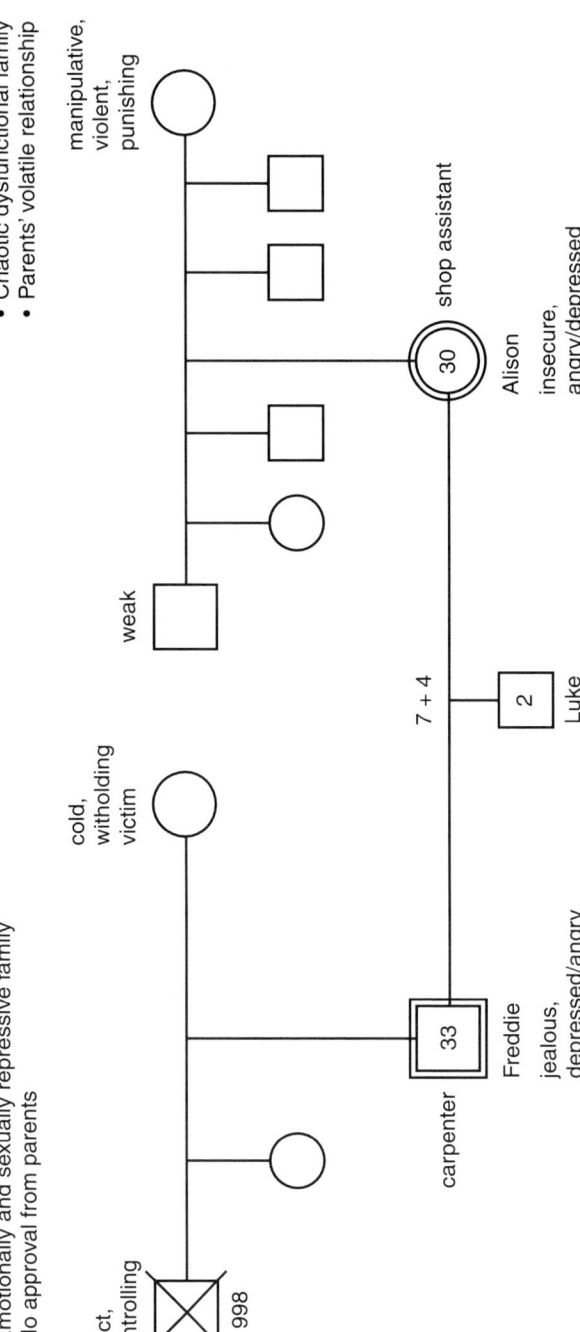

'And baby makes three'

Figure 3.2 'And baby makes three.'

Freddie was 33 and worked as a carpenter. His family was cold and un-emotional; the atmosphere was one of stultifying repression. His father was authoritarian and controlling. His mother told him he was special but with-held affection. He sought parental approval but never got any positive feedback.

Freddie and Alison's relationship had always been stormy but had worsened when Alison got pregnant. Freddie found it difficult to be intimate during her pregnancy. Alison said he let her down during her long and painful labour. Freddie felt jealous and displaced. Alison had doubts about her ability to be a good-enough mother. He was unable to support her as he grew increasingly envious of the attention his son was getting.

Luke's birth was not a joyful event, but a major crisis in the relationship. To add to his difficulties, Freddie's father died soon after Luke was born.

Freddie had been attracted to Alison's warmth and passion. She saw him as calm and strong. But then they discovered each other's hidden shadow side. They both wielded a triumphant destructive power and a need to prove their worthlessness by sabotage.

The projections went deep and they had difficulty separating out what belonged to whom. I felt that in the transference I had to be the strong, con-taining mother who would survive their attacks, who would not be destroyed by their anger or drowned by their depression: the rescuer in the persecution/victim/rescuer triangle.

In the countertransference I felt I was in the presence of two hurt and angry toddlers who cried and shouted and stamped their feet in despair. They were deprived children whose needs could never be met. Luke put them back in touch with their inner wounded child.

If Freddie and Alison could barely be a couple, how could they ever tolerate being a threesome? Freddie was caught in an unresolved Oedipal replay with the arrival of his son. He saw Luke getting all the love and attention that he had missed in infancy and was missing again now. He could not bear the pain of his frustration and envy, which was palpable in the room. Alison barely had enough to sustain her son, let alone Freddie's needs. He threatened to leave the relationship, which terrified Alison.

The status quo was maintained for many months, during which time they both in turn became very depressed. Then Freddie started to separate out and own his projections. He began talking about his sexual needs.

Freddie also carried the ambivalence in the relationship. He was split: part of him wanted to leave the relationship, the fantasy being that his needs could be met elsewhere. Alison was so terrified of being abandoned – she carried his projected fears as well – that she would not easily acknowledge what he was saying.

Talking about physical contact revealed how unlovable they both felt. Alison was ready to give him a little of what he wanted, but he devalued it, and made her feel it would never be good enough. He was punishing her for giving her love to Luke.

I pointed out that sex was the one special thing that he could have with Alison that Luke would never have. He and Luke both had penises but part of resolving the Oedipal issue was knowing that Alison could have his penis but not Luke's. It was hard for Freddie to be in touch with his potency and this had an impact on him. But what he really wanted were Alison's breasts.

He was not just an angry toddler; he was also an infant who did not get the breast when he needed it, resulting in pain, fear, anger, frustration, loss of trust and despair. I saw him as a hungry baby crying alone in a dark room. He was full of revenge and the desire to punish. He was so split that he could only touch Alison if he saw her as an anonymous object.

Because she had become a mother she was no longer a sexual being. He needed her more as a mother than as a sexual partner, which was why the split was maintained. The shared fantasy in marrying was that they would both find a mother in the other.

I had to continue being the loving mother neither of them had had. The longing for intimacy came with great fear because of the terrible grief that ensued if they did not get it. Both needed the other to hold and mother them. Neither was a strong enough container for their fragile egos.

My hope was that in therapy they would find enough ego strength and basic trust to establish some kind of intimacy. Only then could there be any healing. My fear was that their inability to internalise and hold on to any good object would keep them in the status quo: sabotaging the potential to get what they longed for from each other.

■ Affairs

It is becoming increasingly difficult for couples to remain faithful to each other throughout a long-term relationship. Given the rapidly changing social climate, is it possible to remain monogamous for 30, 40 or 50 years? A lot depends on the couple's expectations of themselves and the relationship.

Affairs are a major crisis in relationships. How does one define an affair? Is a one-night stand or a fling an affair? Can one have an affair by email or in a chat-room on the Internet? Does a visit to a massage parlour or a prostitute count as an affair? Does an affair mean sexual intercourse has occurred?

An affair is when one's partner is, or has been, sexually or emotionally involved with a third person.

Affairs are not just a threat to the relationship; they are a sign that there is a problem in the relationship. Many people find themselves attracted to someone else at some point in their relationship, but most of the time they are able to say 'no'. What makes them say 'yes'?

Affairs are often seen as a reason to end a relationship, the *cause* of the break-up. But an affair is usually a *symptom* of something lacking in the relationship, some-thing going wrong. The relationship can recover from an affair if the underlying causes are explored, understood, and steps are taken towards change.

The reasons for having an affair are not just about sex, though sex usually plays a part. Other reasons include:

- lack of attention
- lack of affection
- lack of communication
- not feeling understood
- not feeling valued

- imbalance of power
- boredom
- loneliness
- alienation
- curiosity
- a need for excitement
- a need to rebel
- inability to make a commitment
- fear of intimacy
- a way out of the relationship.

The secrecy of an affair brings risk and a feeling of excitement and naughtiness that goes with illicit activities. It is also an escape into fantasy and 'what if'. But the unfaithful partner is concealing, lying, betraying. There is a serious failure of trust, a degree of separation brought about by the holding of the secret as well as the infidelity.

Disclosure carries its own risks. The betrayed partner will be devastated and will experience many confused feelings similar to bereavement – shock, disbelief, anger, sadness, insecurity, helplessness, powerlessness, loss of self-esteem, shame, failure, despair.

Furthermore, she/he cannot turn to her/his partner for support and consolation in a time of crisis. If the unfaithful partner agrees to end the affair, she/he will also be experiencing loss, grief, guilt and sadness. The betrayed partner will want to know who, when, where, how, what, why. This information will be painful, but not knowing may give rise to fearful fantasies.

If the unfaithful partner has to make a choice, she/he may delay the process, because a decision entails loss, one way or another. It may feel less painful maintaining the status quo.

If the primary relationship is to continue, it will have to be renegotiated on a new basis. Eventually there has to be understanding and forgiveness and a period of rebuilding trust, commitment and intimacy. The problems in the relationship that led to the affair need to be acknowledged, owned and dealt with by both partners if they are to have a shared future with no recurrence of infidelity. This is a daunting task for the couple, who will need the therapy as a safe place to explore the dangerous issues and feelings that are a threat to the relationship itself.

Getting over an affair takes time. The stages are similar to the stages of mourning. Healing comes after resignation, acceptance and letting go.

Example: **'Triangles'**

Ben and Laura had been together for nine years. They had a seven-year-old daughter, Jess, and a son, Charlie, four. The relationship seemed to be a good one, although their intimacy needs were very different. Laura was quite cool and self-contained; Ben was emotional, touchy-feely. Laura avoided confrontation; Ben was more of a volcano. (*See* Figure 3.3.)

Laura's parents had divorced when she was eight and her mother had brought her and her sister up on her own. She was a calm and capable person, whom Laura admired.

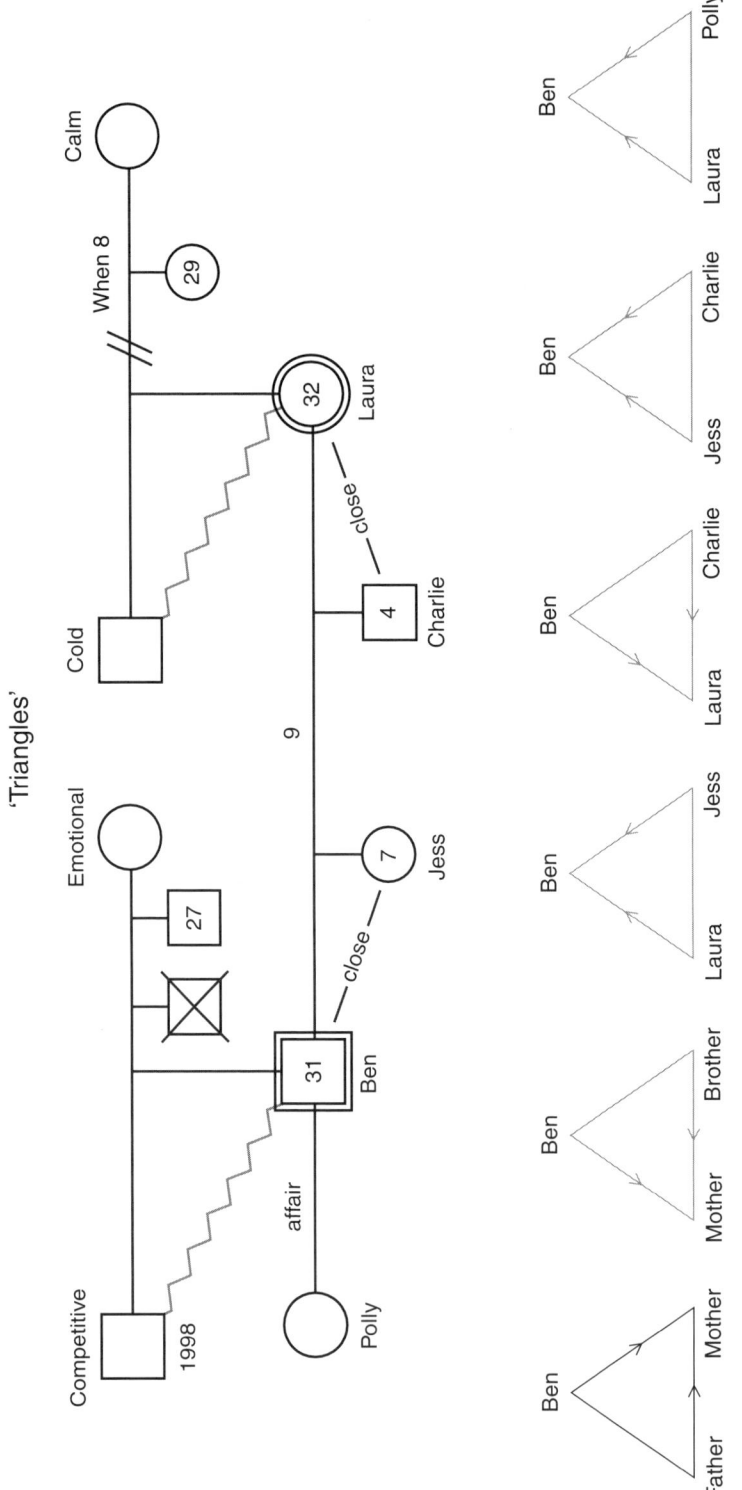

Figure 3.3 Genogram and triangles: Ben and Laura.

Ben was the oldest in his family. The next baby, also a boy, was born prematurely and died soon after his birth. Ben's mother was grief-stricken, but had another baby, also a boy, 18 months later.

In Oedipal terms, Ben must have gone through feelings of jealousy with his lost brother, only to have renewed feelings of jealousy and anger at the birth of the next brother, yet another rival. His relationship with his mother in infancy was confused because she went from joy to grief to joy again, and he went from only child to eldest of two, to only survivor, to eldest of two once more.

Jess was three when Charlie was born. Ben was very close to Jess and was upset by her feelings of jealousy towards her brother. Laura was thrilled to have a son, which somewhat alienated Ben towards the little boy. He also disliked sharing Laura with another male.

By the time his son had turned three, Ben was having an affair. He had identified with the displacement of his daughter and felt excluded by his wife who had been particularly preoccupied with her son. He sought solace and attention with someone else, thereby creating another triangle.

Laura did not want a repeat of her parents' marriage. She could not understand Ben's behaviour: he was the guilty one yet she was being blamed. I was in danger in the transference of becoming the 'other woman'. Ben was in yet another triangle, which felt very familiar. There was a lot of work to do in untangling the family dynamics but first we had to cope with the emotional fall-out of the affair.

■ Separation and divorce

At the time of writing, at least 40% of marriages end in divorce. The figure is near to 60% for second marriages. The figures for long-term relationships most probably exceed these.

Couples dealing with the issue of divorce/separation will present three different agendas:

1 Both have agreed to separate.
2 One wants to end the relationship, the other does not.
3 Neither knows what they want.

When both agree to separate, the work is about a painful ending and the death of the relationship.

When one wants the relationship to end and the other does not, there is an imbalance of power with rejection and abandonment.

When neither knows what they want, ambivalence, uncertainty and maintaining the status quo may be less painful than making a decision and facing loss.

In all three cases, strong, primitive emotions will be experienced. These include:

• confusion
• doubt
• anger
• resentment
• hatred
• fear

- guilt
- shame
- sense of failure
- humiliation
- betrayal
- jealousy
- insecurity
- despair
- violence
- depression.

Therapy with couples where separation is the main agenda can be heavy work because the energy in the room is so negative. The therapist needs to observe her countertransferential reactions and be particularly careful about not taking sides or allowing her personal values to affect the work. Some clients have an idealised fantasy that the therapist will be able to contain their difficult and painful feelings and make the process a smooth and easy one.

Divorce/separation is rarely nice and friendly (unless there is a collusive denial) despite good intentions on both sides. It is partly because the couple have been unable to resolve differences, negotiate successfully and make compromises that they are splitting up. This will be evident in the way they communicate in the consulting room and needs to be reflected back.

Rows, power struggles and battles for control will be acted out and either partner may seek to sabotage the process. The partners may attempt to undermine each other. The therapist needs to work beyond crisis management while keeping the focus on the task in hand and acknowledging how difficult and painful the feelings can be.

A divorce or separation is a major loss and goes through the same stages as bereavement. The danger is that one or other partner may get stuck at the anger or grief stage. Resignation, acceptance and letting go can sometimes take a very long time.

A couple with children will never be able to make a complete, clean break because they will always be parents. This realisation may take time to dawn on them and comes with anger, frustration and disappointment.

Couples will often use money and children as emotional blackmail. If both parents can agree to it, mediation is very helpful in negotiating issues about housing, finances and contact with children. Mediation, however, unlike therapy, does not deal with feelings.

Children do not want their parents to separate. Some couples ask for help in telling their children that they are splitting up. It is not appropriate for the couple's therapist to do family work or give advice, but it may be helpful to let the couple know that children will often feel guilty and to blame. They will need reassurance that both parents love them.

If either of the partners experienced the divorce of their own parents during their childhood, some of the repressed and confused feelings they had then may well surface as the family situation gets repeated.

Ending therapy with a separating couple needs to be handled very sensitively because it is also the end of their relationship. Negative feelings are projected onto the therapist. Frequently couples cancel or do not turn up to the last session because it is too painful. There may be an expectation that one of the partners will continue to see the therapist on their own. This can sometimes invalidate the shared work, as the partner who is leaving may feel that the therapist has been on the other partner's side throughout the process. If in doubt this should be raised in supervision.

There may also be a strong attachment to the therapist, who has carried the last vestiges of hope for the relationship. Clients may regress in a final attempt to hold on to the good mother.

As in all therapeutic work, clients need to be able to integrate what they have learned from the therapist and feel enabled enough to move towards change, both inner and outer.

Like so many events in the life cycle, separation and divorce are about loss. But they can also be about new beginnings.

■ Stepfamilies

It is predicated that by the year 2010 stepfamilies will outnumber nuclear families. The dynamics of the stepfamily are not the same as those of the nuclear family (*see* Figure 3.4).

Couples need to know how a stepfamily will affect their relationship. They will have idealised expectations that are bound to be disappointed.

The hardest role in the extended family is that of step-parent. This is reflected in the myths and stereotypes of the wicked stepmother and the abusive stepfather.

The step-parent comes in as an intruder, an outsider who has not shared much of the family history. The children are often hostile and suspicious. Why should strangers who have been imposed on each other like each other? The natural parent will be split by conflicting loyalties and a desire to make everything all right. There will be rivalry and jealousy, resentment and guilt, which if it is not acknowledged and dealt with will lead to contempt, hatred and a sense of betrayal. Avoidance and denial lead to a veneer of normality over a cauldron of seething emotions.

While the couple are celebrating their new relationship, the children are mourning the disintegration of the original family and the loss of a parent, events over which they had no control. The strongest relationship in the new family is the relationship between the natural parent and the child. The most vulnerable relationship is the couple's. There is no honeymoon phase where they are alone together, just the two of them. Unhappy children will try to gain power and control by manipulative behaviour, emotional blackmail and continuous testing of the boundaries. This leads to an atmosphere of conflict and confrontation, which raises the stress levels.

The stepfamily is a family in transition. The process of becoming a cohesive unit takes a minimum of two years and is marked by confusion, ambivalence and doubt. It is both an emotional and a psychological process, during which everyone has to find a new role. Good communication skills are really important.

The stepfamily needs to go through developmental stages that include restructuring, assimilation and integration. Roles will be redefined, boundaries established. The stages of development in the stepfamily are as follows:

• hopes and fantasies
• mourning the lost family

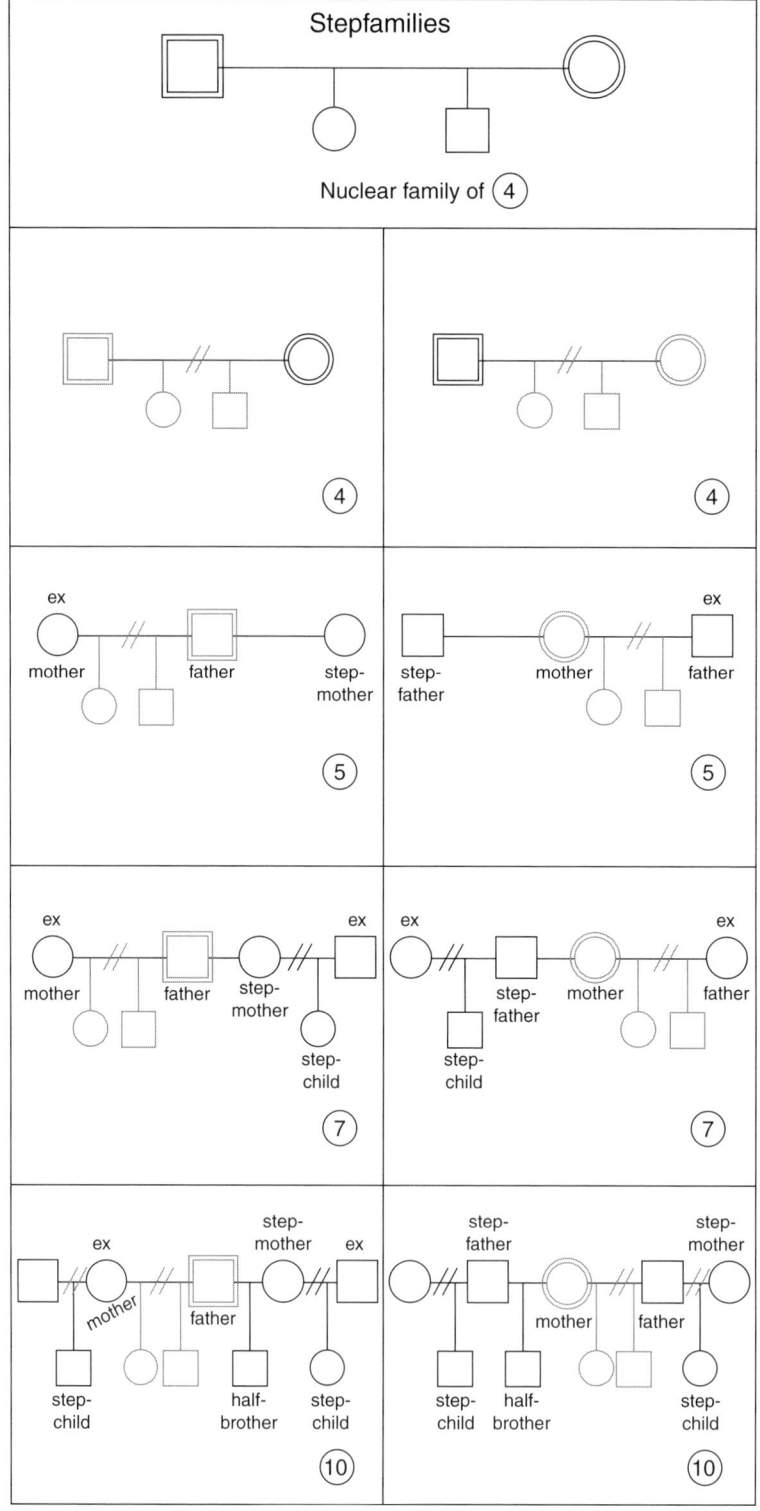

Figure 3.4 Genograms: stepfamilies.

- getting to know each other
- conflicting loyalties, power struggles
- negotiating boundaries and rules
- acceptance and awareness
- integration and moving on.

Discipline and rules will be major issues. Unresolved issues with the ex-partner are likely to surface. The rights and input of the absent parent need to be acknowledged, however difficult for the new couple.

Given the complex interactions of the stepfamily, it is easy for the therapist to get sucked into the system. The focus needs to stay firmly on the couple and their issues. If the therapist is concerned about the children and their relationships to the couple a referral to family therapy might be appropriate.

The following examples show an extended family that failed to make the transition and one that did.

Example: 'Teenage trouble'

Sarah and Roger met at work after Sarah's husband left her. Roger had been divorced for some time. He had two teenage daughters who spent every other week with him. Sarah's children were much younger. Because her house was bigger than his flat, Roger moved in with Sarah. Jessie and Charlotte came to stay on alternate weeks. (*See* Figure 3.5.)

Everything seemed fine at first, because both Roger and Sarah were determined to create one big happy family. Nothing was really discussed, particularly the children's feelings. Everyone was expected to just muddle along.

Sarah had no experience of adolescent girls. She found Roger's daughters strong-willed and dominating, not to mention messy, noisy and temperamental. They did not abide by her rules. She and her children felt invaded. Sarah expected Roger to back her up and was surprised that his loyalties were split. She also discovered to her dismay that he was a very permissive parent.

Her children became quite attached to Roger, although they had little in common with Jessie and Charlotte. He felt that Sarah spoilt them to compensate for their absent father, who was refusing to see them in order to punish Sarah.

Eventually the whole household was competing for Roger's attention. Sarah and Roger needed time and space alone together but were sidetracked by the needs of all the children. There was no unity and they were not operating as a team. They were effectively running two families separately in the same house.

Sarah became the scapegoat and got blamed by everyone for being too controlling. She had wanted to have a baby with Roger in an attempt to bring them closer, but Roger was having doubts about the relationship. His daughters were telling him how tired and unhappy he looked. He and Sarah were rowing a lot.

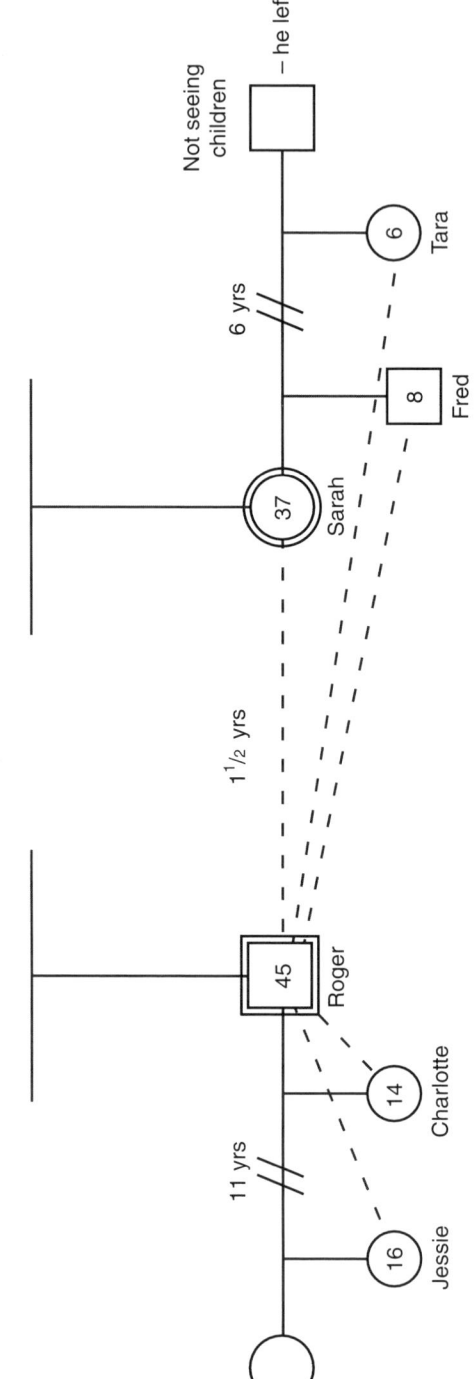

'Teenage trouble'

- All competing for his attention
- She takes all the blame
- Rows
- Different expectations

- One week with mother
- One week with father

Figure 3.5 'Teenage trouble.'

Everything came to a head when Jessie suddenly announced that she did not want to stay there any more and that she would live full-time with her mother. Charlotte was devastated because she felt torn between her sister and her father. Eventually she also left and Sarah realised she was fighting a losing battle. Roger moved out soon afterwards leaving behind two confused and guilty children and Sarah who felt used and abandoned yet again.

Example: **'His, hers and theirs'**

Fiona met Dan five years after her husband had died in a car crash. Her daughter Beth was seven. (*See* Figure 3.6.)

Dan was separated from his wife and had three children, Hugh, Molly and Guy. They visited him every other weekend and for half the school holidays.

Fiona had the good sense to understand that she and Beth were used to being alone together and that Beth did not want to share her. They talked about this and Fiona made sure that she and her daughter had some time to themselves when the other children were staying.

Having lost her father, Beth attached quickly to Dan, who gave her as much attention as he could without upsetting his own children. She was a quiet child who liked to read. His children were sporty and bouncy. Hugh ignored Beth, which suited her. Molly saw her as a rival and did not get close to her. Guy, who had always been treated as the baby, was thrilled to gain a new sister. Beth enjoyed her role of older sister and they became firm friends.

Fiona understood that Dan's children's primary relationship was with him, and gave them the space they needed to sort out the dynamics. She and Dan supported each other over discipline and house rules and managed to be consistent most of the time. There were arguments and tantrums and shouts of 'It's not fair, mummy lets us …', but they stood firm.

Eventually the children grew to like and trust Fiona. She paid attention to them and listened to them. Her way of doing things was not always what they were used to, but they learned to cope with the differences.

The most difficult relationship was with Dan's ex-wife who felt jealous and threatened by Fiona. She was not always co-operative over arrangements for the children. Fiona managed to handle her anger and Dan was supportive without being intrusive.

By giving each other space and by being tolerant and understanding the complexities of the relationships in their extended family, Fiona and Dan managed their own relationship satisfactorily.

Seven years into the relationship, Fiona discovered that she was unexpectedly pregnant. The thought of starting all over again dismayed her and Dan at first, but by the time their son was born, the whole family was enthusiastic and he was a much-loved addition.

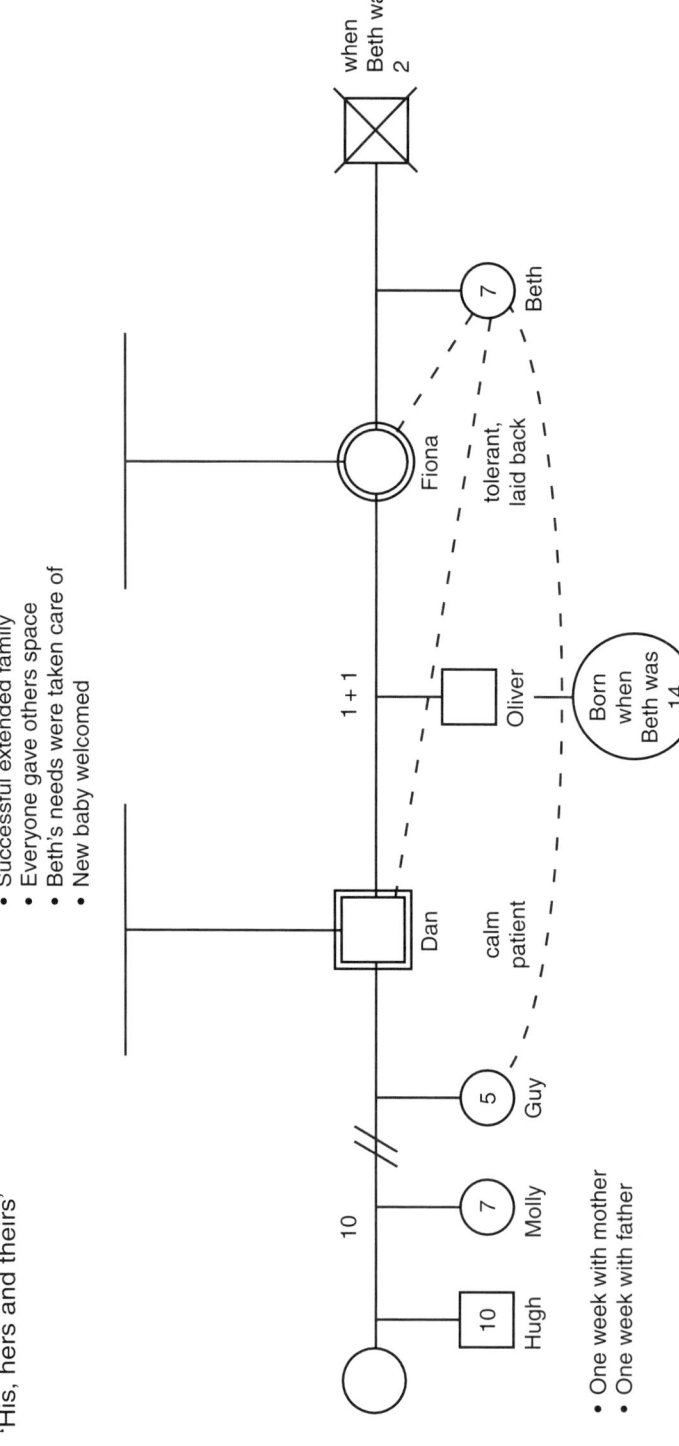

Figure 3.6 'His, hers and theirs.'

■ The mid-life crisis and onwards

Most couples presenting for therapy are in their thirties and forties, with all the issues that come with relationships, families and careers. Part of their problem is that they do not have time to reflect on their lives, especially their inner lives. They project their anxieties and stress onto each other and onto external events. Being busy and working hard are acceptable defences until something cracks – often the relationship, which is taken for granted and not prioritised.

There is a commonly held view that the mid-life crisis is predominantly a male event, which can occur either side of 40. There is an awareness of no longer being immortal, a loss of purpose and energy, a questioning about the meaning of life. This is often expressed in feelings of anxiety, confusion, isolation, alienation, depression and loss of libido. The realisation that half one's life is over and there are ambitions and fantasies that will probably never be fulfilled hits hard. The mid-life crisis is not exclusively a male preserve.

The psychological task is to accept and come to terms with the inevitable disappointments and to continue the journey of transformation with some insight and self-awareness.

On the positive side, this is also a time of productivity and stability, a chance to consolidate one's successes, to reap the rewards both personally and professionally, and to explore new activities that are more appropriate than Harley-Davidsons and sky-diving.

Relationships inevitably come under scrutiny. One may feel trapped by a demanding or distant partner, ageing parents and adolescent children.

Some men will project blame outwards on to the relationship and will act out by having an affair. The lover is often experienced as the longed-for soul-mate who instinctively understands him. She may be a younger woman, who in proving his potency will protect him from the fear of death. The mother/Madonna/whore sexual split may reassert itself.

Women's experience of mid-life crisis is not at all abstract. It is grounded in the physical reality of the menopause, which can take as long as five years, and usually occurs between 45 and 55.

The menopause confirms that a woman's fertility is over. With it come various aspects of physical decline and the fear of loss of status in the outside world. However, the post-war generation, with increasing well-being, longevity and standard of living, are the pioneers of a new model: active, independent, strong, sexual women who are successfully running families, households and careers. If their partners can share their renewed energy and interests, the relationship can move on through the mid-life period with increased stability and enjoyment.

■ The later years

At the moment couples over 60 seldom present for therapy. However, this is likely to change as the social and psychological climate continues to evolve. This pioneering generation, with its high expectations and low tolerance of failure, is likely to seek more help from therapists when relationships between partners are no longer good enough.

This final life stage is ultimately concerned with accepting the inevitability of death and making the most of one's life in the meantime. Coming to terms with one's own mortality is hard and many people choose to stay in denial.

However, it can be a time of freedom and less responsibility. Hopefully one has gained in experience and wisdom, yet is still able to participate actively in life with a degree of serenity and detachment.

If one is continuing to struggle with unresolved issues it may be a time of despair and isolation instead of acceptance and integration. It is all too easy, when faced with physical and cognitive decline, to fall into depression and withdrawal.

The task for couples who have been together for 25 years and more is to let go of old conflicts and resentments, reconcile the past, present and future, and come to terms with what has been, what is and what can be.

Couples can maintain a sexual relationship into their eighties. The nature of their sexual activity may change and be more focused on intimacy and fondness. Mutual support and empathy will help to maintain fulfilment. Good communication is essential.

When the children have left home and the parenting tasks are completed, the couple come face to face, alone together again. Long-term collusions may come under threat or the couple may settle into a defensive system.

Repressed feelings and conflicts may surface again. Men often become more dependent and feel insecure, with a loss of self-confidence. Women, on the other hand, with the knowledge that statistically they will probably outlive their partners, often grow in confidence and independence and continue to maintain an active social life.

Couples who drift apart, and who have less and less in common, may continue to live together out of habit and convenience, silent but separate.

Mutually dependent couples who bicker constantly will cling to each other out of fear and loneliness. When both partners feel nothing but indifference for each other, or the relationship has finally burnt out and feels like an empty shell, separation may be a liberation.

With less social and moral pressure to stay together, a growing number of couples in their fifties and older are choosing to divorce or separate and to continue the end of their journey with a new partner or on their own.

CHAPTER 4

Process

■ Assessment

The aims and objectives of assessment with couples are the same as those of assessment with individuals, but there are extra elements. It is important to keep in mind that in couples therapy it is the relationship between the partners that is the 'client' and that the therapeutic alliance is with the *couple* (*see* Figure 4.1).

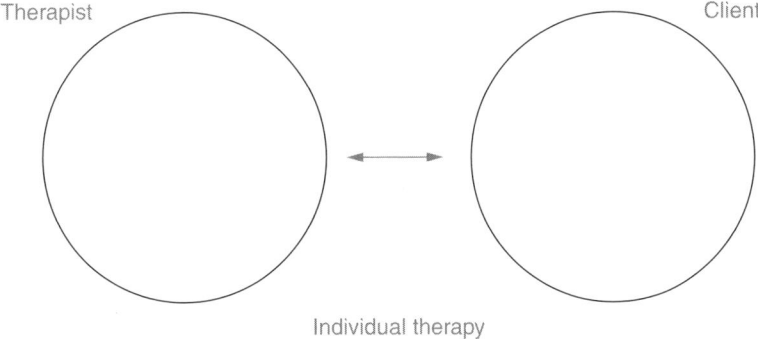

Individual therapy

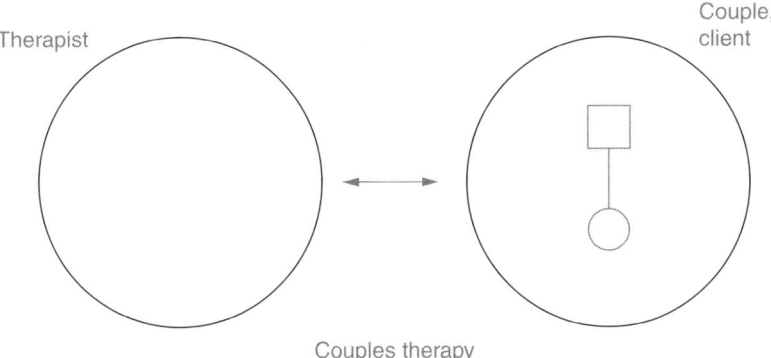

Couples therapy

Figure 4.1   The therapeutic alliance.

An assessment is about gaining and giving information, looking for identifying issues and conflicts, looking at expectations and goals, contextualising the problem and ensuring that the referral is appropriate. It is also about offering a place of safety and containment where neither partner will feel favoured or judged.

The assessment process continues over the first few sessions to include formulation and focus.

The assessment model for couples has three stages:

1 Presenting problem.
2 History of the relationship.
3 Contract.

However, important information will be disclosed about the couple before the first question is asked and in observing their interaction throughout the session.

- Who made the appointment?
  This could be about motivation, who is in charge, who makes the decisions, who is pro-active.
- Who comes in first, who sits down where?
  A chance to look at their appearance, body language, facial expressions, eye contact.
- Who speaks first?
  Does she/he talk from 'I', 'you' or 'we'? Does the partner listen or interrupt? Is there an attempt for one to dominate the session?

■ Presenting problem

Ask each partner in turn to describe what they think is the main problem from their own point of view. Find out how long they have had this problem.

When did things first go wrong?

Why have they decided to ask for help at this particular moment?

This may be connected to an external life event or crisis that has been a triggering factor, or it may be because of a psychological or emotional factor that has tipped the balance.

It is useful to ask each partner for examples of the presenting problem. They may have different perceptions.

Of course, clients come with many problems in their relationship. But the one that they name first is both a conscious and unconscious message about their primary concerns. For example, a couple may say that they argue all the time. The therapist may get into all sorts of material to do with projected anger, power struggle, family history, anxieties and fears.

However, the couple originally intimated that they did not know how to communicate without arguing. Sometimes it is very useful to return to their first words as a focus for the work, particularly when the therapy becomes stuck.

■ History of the relationship

Ask each partner how they met and what attracted them to each other.

Find out what changed and when. There may be a connection to a life event.

Ask them about their sexual relationship, past and present.

See if you can get an overview of their family history.

You need to know about any medical problems and treatment and what previous experience of therapy or counselling they may have had, individually or together.

Knowing their professional occupations will give you an idea of the world they each operate in.

■ Contract

Dates, times and frequency of appointments will need to be negotiated, as well as information about fees, cancellings, missed sessions and breaks.

It is essential when working with couples to make it crystal clear that you will not enter into any telephone, written or email communications with either of them and that you will only see them together as a couple.

Remind them that the relationship between them is the 'client' in the context of couples therapy.

Confirm that your role is not to save their relationship or encourage them to split up.

Let them know that you will work with no blame, no partiality, no judgement. Fault is not an issue.

Make sure that they have fully understood the boundaries and that their expectations of the process are realistic.

It is worth checking how they each feel about your gender as one of them will be outnumbered.

■ Questions in the first session

Throughout the assessment process the therapist will be observing and noting many different factors. She will be asking herself certain questions, checking her assumptions, and using her intellectual deductions as well as her intuition.

These questions, which will generally be unspoken at this point, include the following:

- What is the quality of the couple's interaction?
- Who is labelled 'the problem'?
- Is there blame and accusation or can each of them own their part of the problem?
- Are they coming in crisis? Will either of them be likely to act out?
- Is either of them addicted to alcohol or drugs?
- Is either of them chronically or severely mentally ill or suicidal?
- Have they been instructed to attend by a court, GP or the social services?
- What are their levels of awareness and insight?
- Are they each able to make and maintain an attachment?
- Do they each have sufficient concern for self and others?

- At what levels can they tolerate ambivalence and frustration?
- Do they have the capacity for change?
- Are their agendas similar or opposing?
- What are their expectations of the process?
- What use can they make of the process?
- Can they make a commitment to the process?

Obviously the therapist will not be able to find answers to all these questions in the first session, but it is useful to keep them in mind as part of the assessment process.

Last but not least, in coming to some hypothesis about the couple and their relationship the therapist needs to hold in mind both the transference and the countertransference.

The assessment session is a vital part of creating a positive therapeutic alliance.

It is also extremely useful for the therapist further down the line to refer back to. Not only are all the problems there, so are the answers.

■ The assessment model

Figure 4.2 summarises the three-part assessment model.

■ Formulation and focus

In order to get to the core issues with couples who present for joint therapy it is necessary to move from assessment to formulation. There will inevitably be so much material that it is easy to get waylaid, bogged down or distracted. It is unrealistic to expect to be able to sort out all their issues. The therapist needs to feed this back to the couple and work with them in finding a focus.

Couples will come with individual and shared baggage. It cannot all be unpacked and examined in detail.

In coming to a formulation, the therapist needs to have the following in mind:

- the marital fit
- Oedipal issues
- projective identification
- life-stage events
- the sexual relationship
- the balance between intimacy and autonomy
- communication level and skills
- power and control
- anger and conflict management
- problem solving
- decision-making process
- ability to cope with ambivalence
- capacity for change
- ability to work with difference.

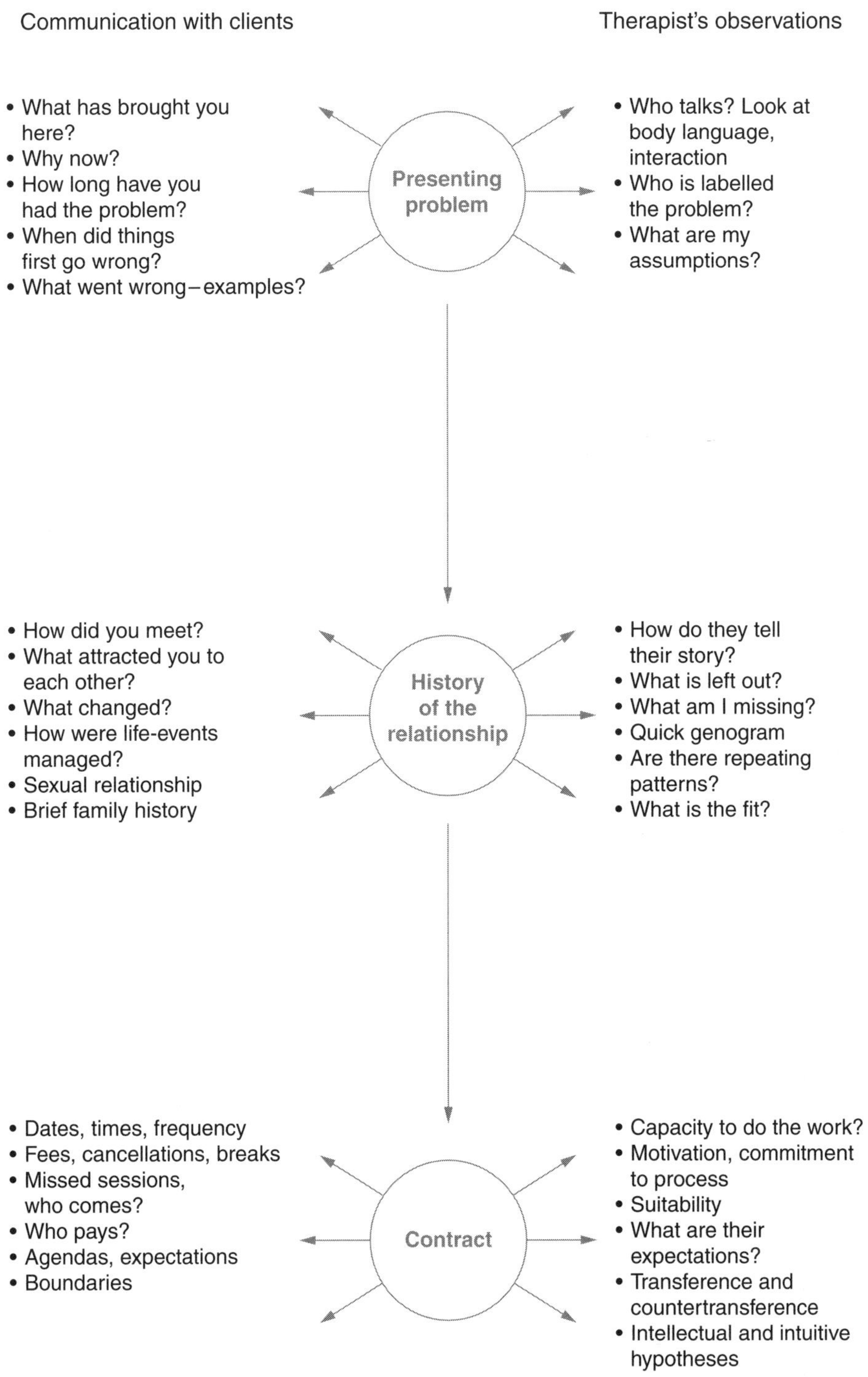

Communication with clients   Therapist's observations

• What has brought you
  here?
• Why now?
• How long have you
  had the problem?
• When did things
  first go wrong?
• What went wrong–examples?

Presenting problem

• Who talks? Look at
  body language,
  interaction
• Who is labelled
  the problem?
• What are my
  assumptions?

• How did you meet?
• What attracted you to
  each other?
• What changed?
• How were life-events
  managed?
• Sexual relationship
• Brief family history

History of the relationship

• How do they tell
  their story?
• What is left out?
• What am I missing?
• Quick genogram
• Are there repeating
  patterns?
• What is the fit?

• Dates, times, frequency
• Fees, cancellations, breaks
• Missed sessions,
  who comes?
• Who pays?
• Agendas, expectations
• Boundaries

Contract

• Capacity to do the work?
• Motivation, commitment
  to process
• Suitability
• What are their
  expectations?
• Transference and
  countertransference
• Intellectual and intuitive
  hypotheses

Figure 4.2   The assessment model.

ACT: Are they able to:

- **Accept**
- **Compromise**
- **Tolerate?**

When the process gets stuck, because change is too threatening, the therapist can challenge the couple as follows.

> 'You have three choices:
> 1 Nothing changes, in which case the status quo actually suits you. Accept the situation, embrace the pain, move on.
> 2 There has to be change because the status quo is unbearable. You agree to separate and move on.
> 3 Neither of you want to stick with the status quo or separate. There has to be change. You can't make your partner change; you can only make changes in yourself.'

Any one of these challenges will provide a focus for the work. The couple have also been reminded that they have to do the work. The therapist, who may hold the hope, cannot do it for them. There is no magic wand.

■ Counselling model

The counselling model incorporates assessment, formulation and focus (*see* Figure 4.3).

■ What happens if ...?

- Only one person turns up to the session.
  Explain that you agreed to always see them as a couple and you cannot see her/him on her/his own.
- One person is late.
  Explain that you cannot start the session until the partner arrives.
- One person speaks for both of them.
  Ask them to speak from the 'I' position, not 'you' or 'we'.
- One person dominates the session.
  Reflect this back to them and facilitate the other person's participation.
- They have a huge row in the session.
  Reflect back that it is OK and safe to do that. Make sure you can contain them.
- One person storms out of the room.
  Tell the remaining person that you cannot continue the session with her/him, but that you will be available to them as a couple until their time is up.
- Both attack you verbally.
  Reflect back their anger and do not allow yourself to be de-skilled.
- One person threatens violence to her/his partner or to you.

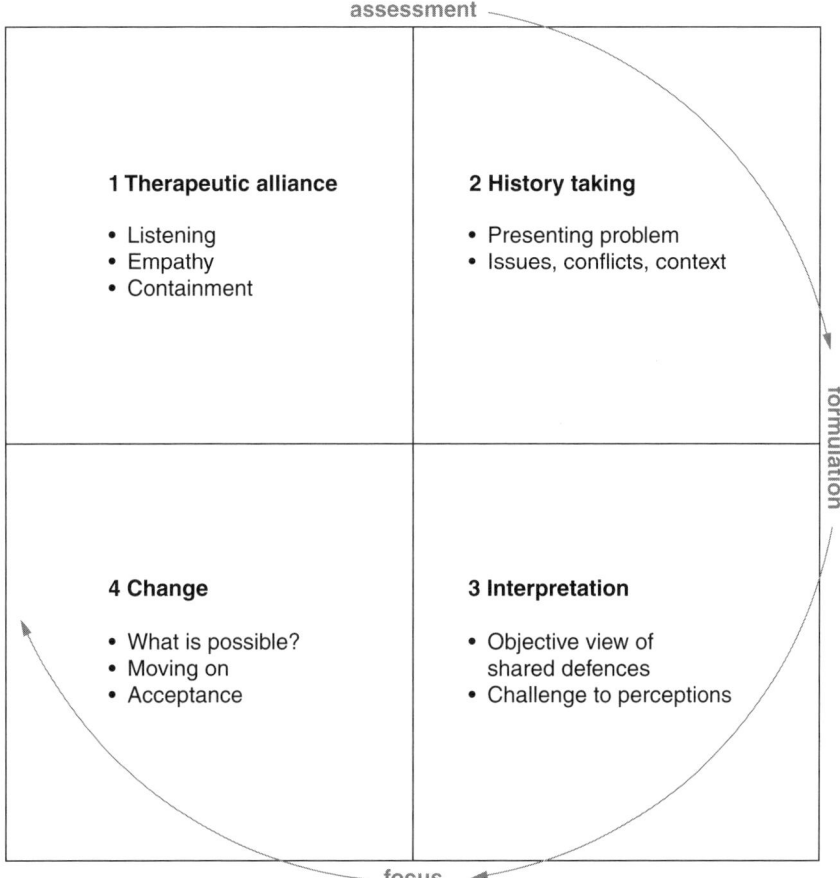

Figure 4.3 The counselling model.

Make it very clear that violence in your consulting room is unacceptable. If the violent person stands up, stand up too so that you are at equal levels. Leave the room if you feel seriously threatened.

- One person drops a bombshell or betrays a secret.
  Be professional. Do not react in shock or surprise. Be aware of the level of manipulation. Be prepared for the consequences.
- They compete for your attention.
  Reflect this back. Look for repeating triangular patterns and situations in their relationship. Do not take sides. Be objective.
- One of them attempts to ally themselves with you against the other.
  Reflect this back and explore it with each of them. Do not collude.
- They come with completely different agendas.
  See if there is any room for negotiation, any middle ground. If not, reflect back that that is the reality.
- Neither one is able to accept change.
  Explore what it is about the status quo that is safe and suits them. Look at the anxieties that come with the possibility of change.

- One partner is repeatedly late.
  Look at his/her commitment to the process. Is it unconscious provocation, an expression of anger with their partner or with you? Do you start without her/him?
- There is an issue about paying your fee.
  Do they share the cost? Is it always the same person who pays? Does that person ever forget their cheque book or the cash? Reflect back and explore.
- They come to the session with a breast-feeding baby or a toddler.
  Explain that the infant is a person in its own right whose presence will affect the interaction. Encourage them to make baby-sitting arrangements.
- One person comes with a relative or friend instead of their partner.
  Remind her/him that your contract is with the couple and you cannot see her/him with anyone else.
- A married person comes to the first session with her/his lover.
  This is the presenting couple. Work with their relationship. It would not then be appropriate to see the married couple.
- Only one person is willing to attend.
  Invite the missing partner in with a welcoming letter. Offer her/him an individual session to keep the balance. Stress that their session will be completely confidential. If she/he refuses to attend you can still work very effectively with the attending partner if you keep the focus on the relationship. It is not helpful to invite the missing partner in after the first couple of sessions because by then you will have formed a therapeutic alliance. The partner will see you as a team and will feel excluded.
- Both clients have agreed to separate.
  You are helping them through a bereavement process, which includes anger, sadness, resignation and letting go. There will be loss, grief, a sense of disillusionment, disappointment and failure. There may be bitterness and resentment. Their self-esteem and sense of self-worth will be affected. They may want to explore the history of the relationship in order to understand when and how it went wrong. There will be a shared fantasy that the separation process will be smooth and amicable. If there are children, property and finances to sort out, it may be appropriate to refer them to mediation.
- One partner has decided to end the relationship; the other wants it to continue.
  The partner who wants out is the one with the power. You need to reflect back what you are hearing to the other one, who may be in denial. If the partner who is leaving only attends one or two sessions, it is appropriate to continue working with the abandoned one.
- She is pregnant: one of them wants a termination; the other does not.
  There is obviously an issue about time and a black and white decision to be made. Keep the focus on the relationship, how they communicate, what their hopes and fears may be. Whatever the outcome, there is a strong possibility of resentment and guilt.
- One partner wants to have a baby; the other does not.
  This is another situation where there is no middle way, no compromise that can be negotiated. Again, keep the focus on the relationship. Exploring their own experiences of childhood will be important. When someone has had a difficult, unloved and painful childhood they are often fearful of bringing a child into the world and repeating the experience. Others desperately need to have a child so as to make it different and find some healing.

Working with couples is challenging and exciting. The dynamics and interactions may be unpredictable. They may bring constant crises and dramas as a way of not getting into the real work.

Couples will act out, sabotage and be manipulative, either together or as individuals. This can be extremely informative about the relationship issues. It is important to keep the focus on the relationship and not get sucked in to what may well be diversionary tactics and red herrings.

However, it can be helpful to work through an individual issue in the session because the partner may learn something relevant to the relationship. This needs to be negotiated and equal time offered to the other partner in a subsequent session.

If individual issues come to dominate the session it is worth considering a referral to one-to-one therapy.

If the clients can manage it emotionally, financially and time-wise it is OK for either or both of them to have one-to-one therapy as well as couples therapy.

There is a danger in the transference of a 'good cop/bad cop' split where one therapist is idealised and the other devalued. The individual therapist needs to know that the client is also in couples therapy.

Example: **Alan and Holly – assessment, formulation and focus**

(Throughout this case the therapist's thoughts are given in italics.)

Holly was six months pregnant with her second baby. (*See* Figure 4.4.)

This meant that there would be a break in the therapy and that they would be going through a major life event.

Holly seemed anxious and Alan seemed a little nervous but they were open and easy to talk to and connect with. He was courteous and they responded instinctively to each other.

She came across as an extrovert. Her clothes were colourful. He seemed more conservative, quite reserved, but with a dry humour.

I guessed that they were probably quite different and opposed.

He needed flexibility because he was away a lot on business.

(Was this a possible source of stress?)

Presenting problem

They argued a lot, which left them both feeling bad. She said she felt under-valued, not prioritised. He said his feelings had changed in the last two years and that he had withdrawn from the relationship.

Their first child was two years old. Had he felt undervalued, not prioritised when the baby was born? Was this being projected onto her?

Why now?

The birth of their second baby was coming up. Their son was two. Their family was expanding.

What was their experience of infancy? Did their situation arouse unconscious issues around their position in their own families? Oedipal, rivalry, triangles?

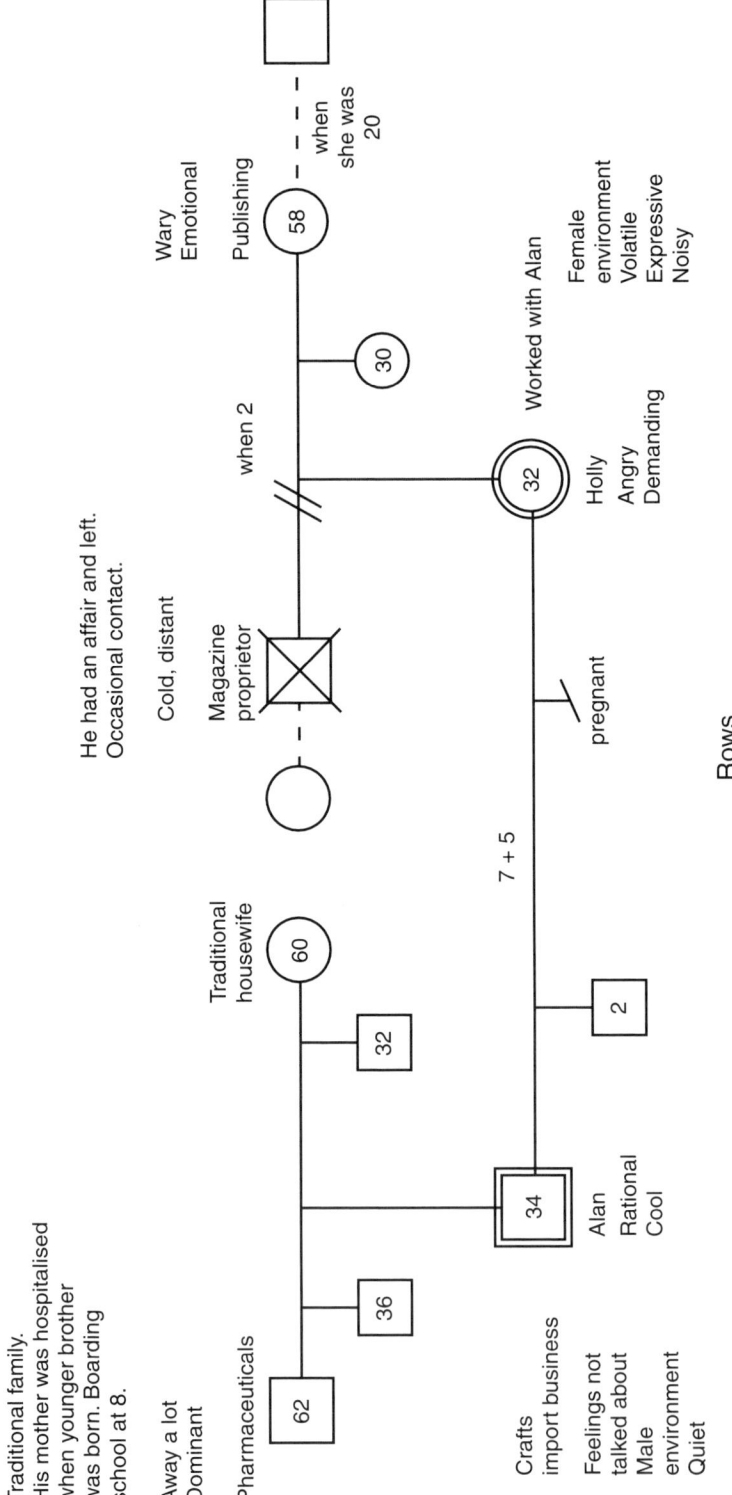

Figure 4.4   Alan and Holly – assessment, formulation and focus.

History of the relationship

Alan and Holly had been together for 12 years and had been married for five years.

They were attracted to each other because they had similar interests and values. He liked her gregarious social nature and her warmth and generosity. She made him feel special.

But not any more.

She felt he would be a responsible and reliable partner who would not let her down.

Was this an idealised fantasy?

They had travelled a lot together and set up a business that imported crafts. Holly's parents had divorced after her sister was born when she was only two.

Was there an unconscious fear of repeating this pattern with the birth of her second child?

Holly had been depressed and anxious for many years. She had depended on Alan who had looked after her. Becoming a mother had helped her to feel much stronger and so she needed him less. There had been a shift in the relationship. Their sexual relationship was satisfactory and both pregnancies had been planned.

Family history

Alan was the middle child of three boys. His father travelled a lot; he described his mother as loyal and traditional. His father was the dominant one. Just after the birth of his younger brother when he was two, Alan's mother was hospitalised for a week and he was effectively 'abandoned'.

Being two years old and the arrival of the next baby were major crises points for both Alan and Holly.

Alan was sent to boarding school at the age of eight and had learned to rationalise and repress his feelings. He idealised his childhood and his family, which irritated Holly.

Holly's background was very different. Her mother, whom she described as warm, emotional and independent, had always worked. She had remarried when Holly was 20. Her father was distant and cold. He had let them all down by leaving. She had grown up in a very female environment. Alan's family was very male.

Formulation

Becoming parents had awakened shared unconscious fears of abandonment and fantasies of being made to feel special and unique.

She was attracted by his united and traditional family and felt that he would take care of her and look after her. She expected him to be 'new man', an equal partner who would share the childcare and domestic arrangements, unlike her father.

He felt displaced by the birth of his son and feared feeling even more excluded with the arrival of the new baby. He had discovered that he did not enjoy being 'new man'; he wanted to be 'traditional man' like his father, the provider and head of the family. And he wanted Holly to be like his mother, loyal and traditional. Now that she was no longer so dependent on him emotionally, he did not feel needed any more.

Their shared, unresolved Oedipal issues manifested in competitive power struggles and battles for control. She projected her anger with her father onto him. He retreated into reason and humour.

Her fear was that Alan would withdraw from the relationship and leave. His fear was that he would be redundant once she had her two babies. Her feeling of not being valued was his projective identification.

They had different experiences and expectations of family life, gender roles, dependence and independence, and the expression of emotions.

Their narcissistic wounds prevented them from empathising with each other's feelings. They each put their own needs first. Their communication was like that of spoilt angry toddlers: 'I want', 'I'm fed up with you', 'It's not fair', 'You're horrible'.

In the transference I was the tolerant and fair mother who would survive their angry and persecutory attacks. In the countertransference I felt like the punishing mother (her) with an urge to withdraw (him).

Focus
With so much material to work with and a break in the process for the birth of the baby, I wanted to keep the focus on the here and now and the previous two years. I explored gender expectations and Oedipal issues and looked at their unconscious fear of repeating patterns.

Outcome
Alan and Holly were unable to make any real changes or compromises. They were destined to repeat her parents' marriage. He decided to leave, she was hurt and angry, both were deeply disappointed. Neither could own their projections.

Had I been a good-enough mother?

■ Transference and countertransference

Classical psychoanalysis attaches very great import and meaning to working with the transference and countertransference. Both have a significant role to play in couples therapy but may be considered as two of the many tools that are useful in understanding the dynamics in the consulting room.

Put in the simplest terms, they may be described as follows.

- *Transference*: Who do we remind the clients of and what feelings does it bring up in them?
- *Countertransference*: Who do the clients remind us of and what feelings does it bring up in us?

Working with the transference and countertransference is about making the unconscious conscious by acknowledging and paying attention to these feelings as they arise.

When there are three people in the room the number of conscious and unconscious messages may seem overwhelming. It would not be feasible to interpret them all. However, certain themes are universal to couples work and merit attention as unconscious communications. These include:

- Oedipal issues
- attachment issues
- gender issues
- alliances
- splits
- competitiveness
- sexual attraction.

Clients may share unconscious expectations of the therapist who may be idealised or devalued in the transference. When the transference is split one client may attempt to side with the therapist and the other will criticise or attack.

Transferential feelings include:

- anger
- envy
- dislike
- power
- control
- love
- idealisation
- erotic
- protective
- intimacy.

When one member of the couple has a positive transference with the therapist and the other a negative transference it is important to acknowledge the split as it represents a difference between the couple as well as the relationship between each of them and the therapist (*see* Figure 4.5).

Working with the countertransference is extremely helpful in understanding what is going on between the couple.

The therapist may take on the role of rescuer, caretaker, nurturer. She may feel omnipotent and wise, expert and all-knowing.

Negative feelings in the therapist include:

- depression
- anger
- helplessness
- anxiety
- discomfort
- dislike
- envy
- frustration
- judgemental
- critical
- persecutory
- arrogant

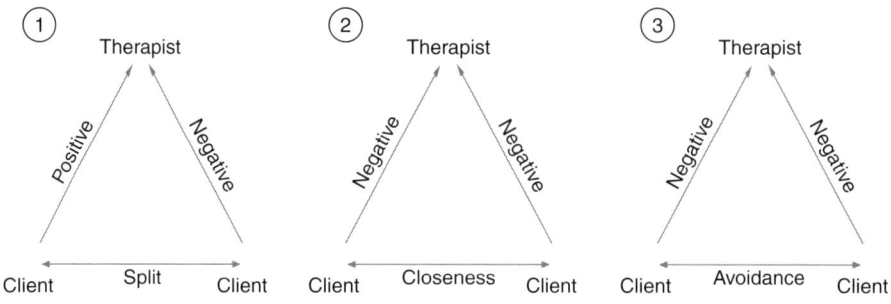

Transference

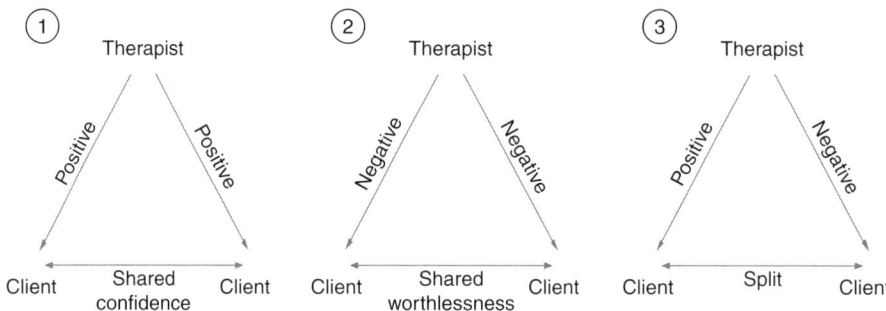

Countertransference

Figure 4.5 Transference and countertransference: triangles.

- powerful
- de-skilled
- useless
- bored.

When these feelings are particularly strong, unusual or unexpected, the therapist needs to pay attention to them, particularly if they apply to one member of the couple.

Is it always useful to investigate the transference and the countertransference? Not necessarily, if this is not the way the therapist usually works. However, as an informative and diagnostic tool it is generally worth examining even if it is not shared in those terms with the clients. (*See* Figures 4.6a and 4.6b.)

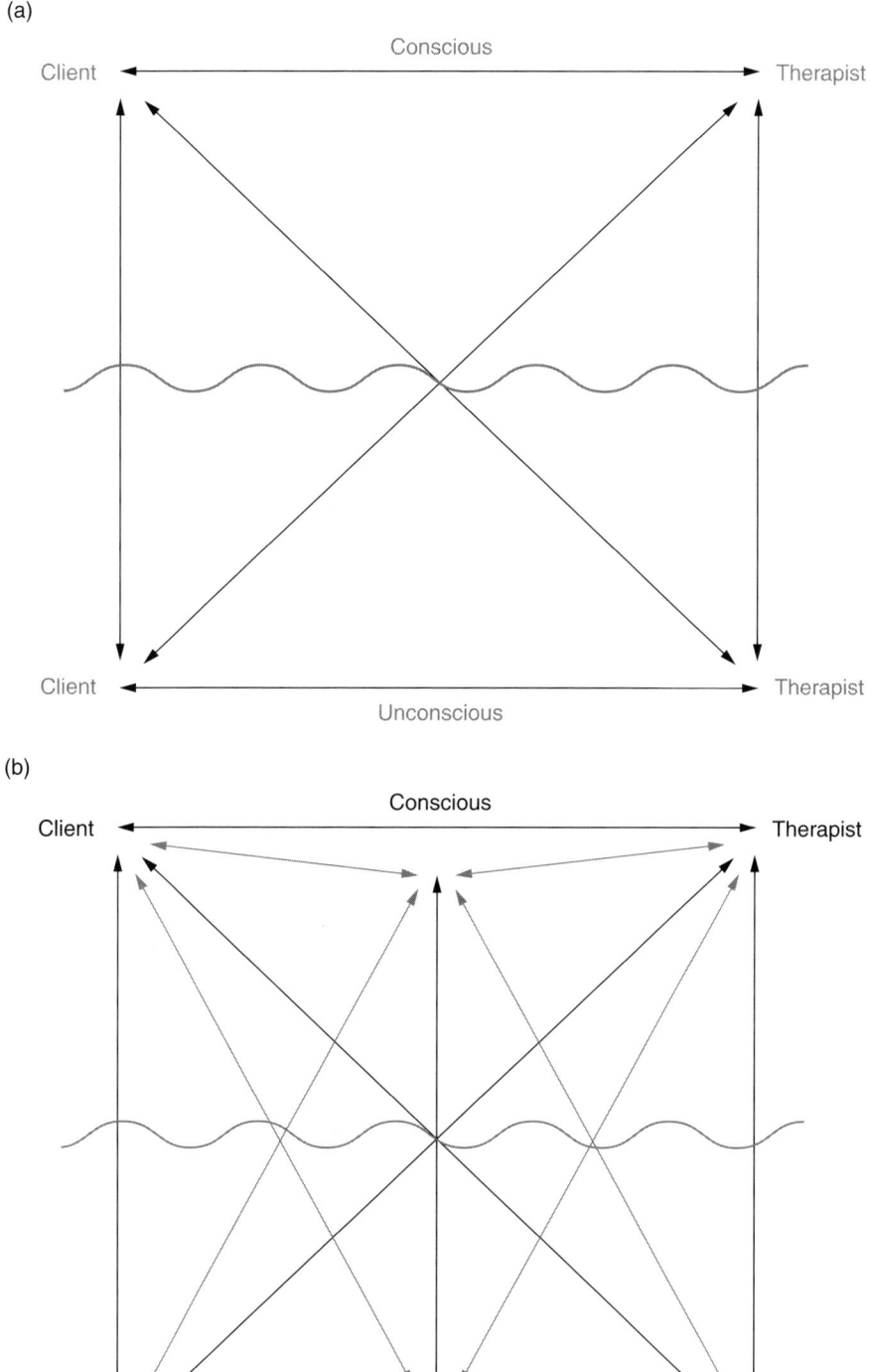

(a)

Conscious

Client   Therapist

Client   Therapist

Unconscious

(b)

Conscious

Client   Therapist

Client   Therapist

Unconscious

'Cat's cradle'

Figure 4.6 Transference and countertransference: (a) individual therapy; (b) couples therapy.

Example: **Steve and Kate** (*see* **Figure 4.7**)

Steve and Kate came to therapy because they were disappointed in their marriage. They had been together for five years and had a little boy of three. Her parents were in a loveless marriage; his father had gone when he was five.

In the first few weeks I took to Kate most warmly – I found her open, expressive and easy to work with. Steve on the other hand seemed very narcissistic and distinctly unsexy – I felt disappointed, just like Kate.

As the work developed, there was a shift. Steve was very eager to please me. In the transference, I was the accepting mother, but in the countertransference I was left strangely angry. When I raised this with him he admitted to feelings of anger not just with his mother but also with Kate. This was the first time he had expressed his anger.

Kate, however, was moving away from me, which irritated me. I found myself colluding with her transferential feelings and was in danger of becoming a critical parent. I did not share this with her. But she revealed that she felt unable to please her parents, who were both critical. This was also how she felt with Steve. He, of course, had not seen himself in that role. Steve had seemed to be the one with the problems, which was a sure sign that Kate was just as damaged.

I started to perceive her as a frightened little girl who did not ever feel good enough. I was able to respond as a nurturing mother.

Meanwhile, Steve reverted to being passive. I had to encourage him to stay in touch with his feelings. Eventually, they both started to feel better about themselves and more confident with each other.

Interestingly, Steve had initially appeared unsexy to me but it was Kate who had lost her desire. Because he felt sexually rejected, he had switched off, which I had picked up.

Working with the transference and countertransference was only one aspect of the therapy with Kate and Steve, but it was informative and valuable in understanding their dynamic, particularly when it started to shift (*see* Figure 4.8).

■ Personal issues

It is important for the therapist to acknowledge that her personal beliefs, values, social and cultural background may be different from those of the couple. This is particularly relevant to relationships and how the couple choose to conduct theirs.

The therapist also needs to be aware of parallels in her own life and relationship. These may be present in the following areas:

- pregnancy
- children
- parenting
- sex

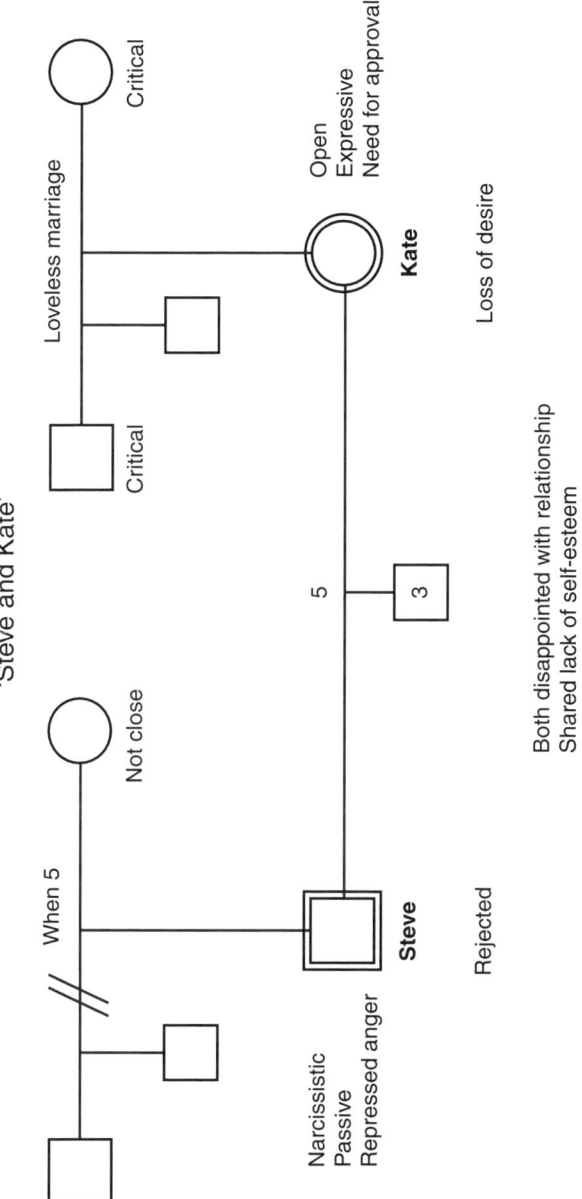

Figure 4.7 Genogram: Steve and Kate.

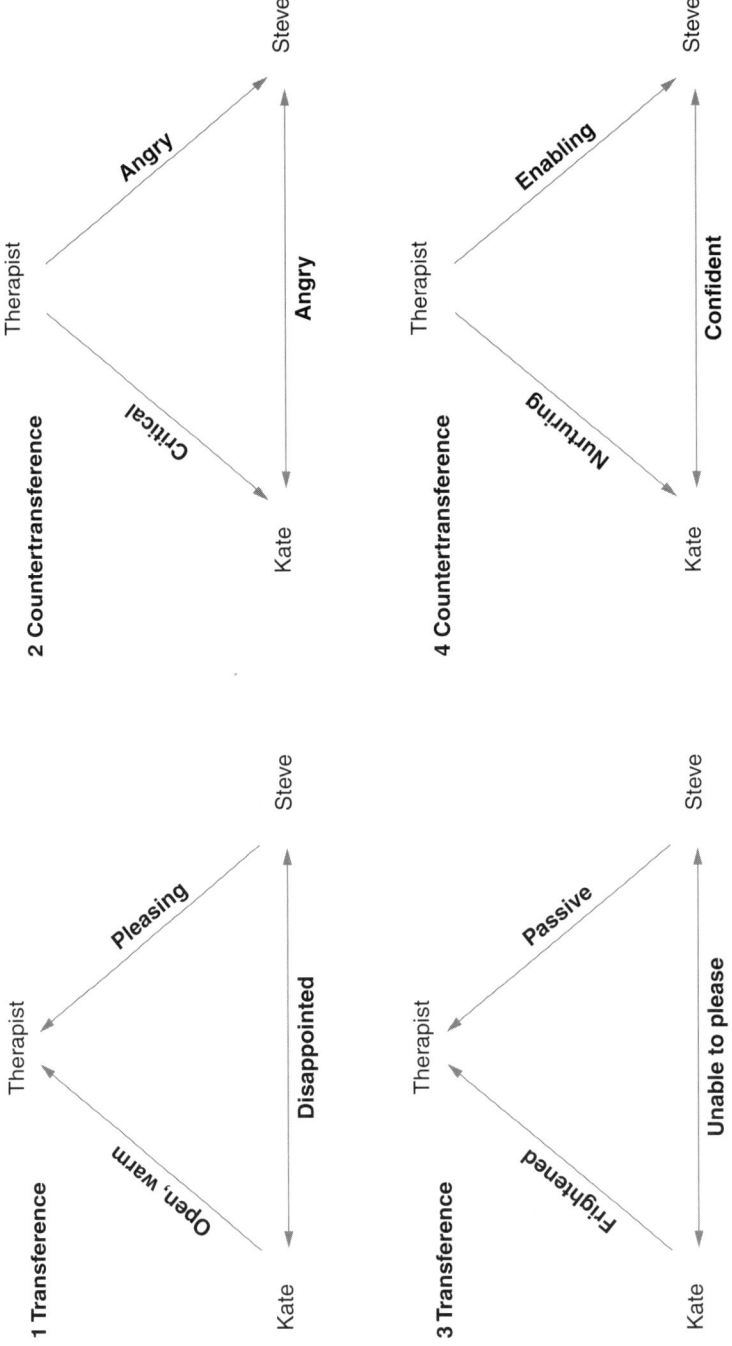

Figure 4.8 Transference and countertransference: Steve and Kate.

- affairs
- divorce
- money
- careers
- illness
- death
- bereavement
- other life events
- unexplored issues.

If the therapist is seriously troubled by countertransferential issues, she needs to raise them in supervision or in personal therapy. The therapist needs to keep firm boundaries, particularly around disclosure, as this could give rise to envious fantasies.

■ Erotic transference and countertransference

This is an area of psychotherapeutic work which is avoided, denied or repressed because to acknowledge sexual feelings in the room could put the clients and the therapist in touch with embarrassment, discomfort, guilt, shame, curiosity, desire, voyeuristic or lustful fantasies.

It is easy to fall into a comfortable collusion and simply not raise the issue. This would miss an important part of the work, particularly in couples therapy. Sexual transference and countertransference carry meaningful messages about the dynamics of the clients' relationship.

Looking at the reasons for the collusion is also informative because it reflects the collusion between the couple.

Erotic transference (from the client to the therapist) is often about an unconscious longing to be merged. Being in love puts one back in touch with the merging of mother and baby. Sex is the vehicle in adults that can lead to this feeling of merging.

In the countertransference the therapist becomes a maternal rescuer or erotic partner. Therapists need to feel valued, but flattery, flirting and seduction, though sometimes tempting, are not the best way.

By acknowledging the client's erotic transference the therapist makes it safe for the client to get in touch with her/his unconscious fantasies. It also makes her/his sexuality containable and acceptable. The therapist can explore why the client is using sexuality as a means of communication, whether it is a pattern of behaviour and what it may symbolise.

In couples work the erotic transference will provide clues as to what is going on between the clients, who is carrying what for whom, who is acting out and why it may suit the other partner.

The primitive libidinal material is repressed because it is too risky for the client to make it conscious to her/his partner so it is acted out in the consulting room between the client and the therapist.

This triangulation is often a replay of the Oedipal situation. The client is in an 'affair' with the therapist. The partner may have strong feelings of rivalry, envy and jealousy because the therapist is sharing something special and intimate with the client. She is also enabling and empowering the client. The partner's role is being usurped.

Erotic countertransference in the therapist does not have to be made explicit in the work, but the therapist needs to own it and separate what is her material and what belongs to the clients.

This is not always easy. The therapist may feel attracted and turned on. Intense sexual fantasies may arise. These may resonate with some private experience in her past and not have anything to do with the client. Self-awareness is crucial.

The therapist may have erotic thoughts, feelings or dreams outside the sessions. Something is going on in the process that has touched her unconscious.

If the therapist has an intense curiosity or voyeuristic fantasies about the couple's sexual relationship this is more likely to be about what is or is not going on between the couple. It may not even be about sex; it may symbolise some other form of connection or communication.

The therapist may feel she is in a position of power and authority. Clients are often dependent and vulnerable.

It is absolutely essential that the therapist behaves professionally and ethically. The boundaries must be observed. If the therapist feels in danger of acting out, this needs to be explored in supervision.

Therapy, like sex, is an intense experience. There needs to be a delicate balance in the work between caution and risk. We need to be attentive, intuitive and open. We need to work with love, not sex.

Further reading

- Abel-Hirsch N (2001) *Eros (Ideas in Psychoanalysis)*. Icon Books, Cambridge.
- Beattie M (1997) *Co-dependent No More*. Hazelden Information and Educational Services, USA.
- Cashdan S (1988) *Object Relations Therapy: using the relationship*. WW Norton, New York.
- Cleese J and Skynner R (1993) *Families and How to Survive Them*. Vermilion, London.
- Clulow C and Mattinson J (1995) *Marriage Inside Out: understanding problems of intimacy*. Penguin Books, London.
- Dicks HV (1993) *Marital Tensions: clinical studies towards a psychological theory of interaction*. Karnac Books, London.
- Dowling E and Barnes G (1999) *Working with Children and Parents through Separation and Divorce. The Changing Lives of Children* (Basic Texts in Counselling and Psychotherapy). Palgrave-Macmillan, Basingstoke.
- Engel B (2002) *The Emotionally Abusive Relationship*. John Wiley, Chichester.
- Gilbert M and Schmukler D (1996) *Brief Therapy with Couples*. John Wiley, Chichester.
- Gray J (2002) *Men are from Mars, Women are from Venus*. HarperCollins, London.
- Hendrix H (2001) *Getting the Love You Want: a guide for couples*. Henry Holt, New York.
- Hildebrand P (1995) *Beyond Mid-life Crisis: a psychodynamic approach to ageing*. Sheldon Press, London.
- Jacobs M (1998) *The Presenting Past: the core of psychodynamic counselling and therapy*. Open University Press, Buckingham.
- Johnson R (1988) *The Psychology of Romantic Love*. Penguin Books, London.
- Katzenberg S (1999) *I Want a Divorce?* Kyle Cathie, London.
- Laing RD (1998) *Knots*. Routledge, London.
- Litvinoff S (1998) *Relate Guide to Better Relationships: practical ways to make your love last*. Vermilion, London.
- McGoldrick M (1999) *Genograms, Assessment and Intervention*. WW Norton, New York.
- Norwood R (1989) *Women Who Love Too Much*. Arrow, London.
- Pincus L and Dare C (1980) *Secrets in the Family*. Faber and Faber, London.
- Robinson M and Smith D (1993) *Step by Step: focus on stepfamilies*. Harvester Wheatsheaf, Hemel Hempstead.
- Ruszczinksi S (1993) *Psychotherapy with Couples*. Karnac Books, London.
- Scarf M (1987) *Intimate Partners: patterns of love and marriage*. Century Hutchinson, London.
- Scharff D and Scharff J (1995) *Object Relations Couple Theory*. Jason Aronson, New Jersey.

- Sharp D (1998) *The Survival Papers: anatomy of a midlife crisis*. Inner City Books, Toronto.

- Skynner R (1976) *One Flesh: Separate Persons. Principles of Family and Marital Psychotherapy*. Constable and Robinson, London.

- Solomon M and Siegel J (eds) (1997) *Countertransference in Couples Therapy*. WW Norton, New York.

- Tannen D (1992) *You Just Don't Understand: women and men in conversation*. Virago, London.

- Wallerstein J and Blakeslee S (1996) *The Good Marriage: how and why love lasts*. Bantam, London.

- Willi J (1996) *Couples in Collusion*. Jason Aronson, New Jersey.

- Winnicott D (1991) *The Child, the Family and the Outside World*. Penguin Books, London.

- Young R (2001) *The Oedipus Complex (Ideas in Psychoanalysis)*. Icon Books, Cambridge.

PART 2

Sex

CHAPTER 5

Good sex

■ The meaning of sex

We live in a society that emphasises sexuality, sex appeal and sexual gratification. All kinds of pornography are available on the Internet to satisfy our fantasies. The media bombard us with images and messages that raise our expectations to an unrealistically high level.

In opposition to this are the cultural and religious dictates that have prevailed for centuries and have created guilt, fear and shame in generation after generation. The sexual revolution of the 1960s is recent history but the feminist movement and the Pill have led to huge changes in society, some of which have caused new confusion and anxiety, particularly with regard to gender roles.

While new man and post-feminist woman are trying to work out a more equal sexual relationship, macho man and traditional woman are still alive and well out there – if increasingly unsure about how to conduct their love lives.

How important then is sex in a couple's relationship? What is sex for? What does it mean to each of them? What are their expectations about quality and quantity? These are questions that couples need to be able to address in their relationship.

A fulfilling sexual relationship gives a couple a shared feeling of self-worth and validation, confirmation and unity. A long-lasting sexual relationship needs intimacy and commitment, but it also needs imagination and creativity to keep it from becoming stale.

The essence of sex is about merging and fusing, both physically and emotionally, spiritually even. This can be risky. One needs to be able to let go and lose control, to allow oneself to be utterly open and vulnerable with one's partner in absolute safety. Good sex in a long-lasting relationship is primarily about mutual trust and respect. Chemistry and good technique are not enough in themselves.

The intense and passionate honeymoon phase in a relationship can last for months or even years. But it is not realistic to believe it will continue in that way for decades. At some point the couple have to move from being 'in love' to 'loving'. Sex needs to transform into something more peaceful, comfortable and familiar. It can signify an even more binding and profound relationship, based on mutual trust and a greater knowledge of the other partner as they really are and not as the idealised figures that each first appeared to be. Some people find it very hard to move from 'in love' to 'loving'. They are hooked on the excitement, the rush, the buzz of sex. They want the thrill to go on forever and will use phrases such as 'The spark has gone' or 'It's not as exciting as it used to be' or 'I don't fancy her/him any more'.

Moving from illusion to disillusion and coming to terms with reality can be hard, painful even. Many will give up on the relationship and look for a new sexual partner, embarking on serial monogamy. Or they will have affairs, flings or one-night stands to keep the adrenaline going.

The meaning and purpose of sex are many and various. Some of the feelings associated with good sex include:

- love
- pleasure
- fun
- thrill
- excitement
- lust
- intimacy
- comfort
- reassurance
- bonding
- communion
- tenderness
- security
- passion
- transcendence
- power
- control
- well-being.

Good sex may be described as:

- erotic
- satisfying
- relaxing
- gentle
- sensual
- primitive
- energetic
- emotional
- intense
- mystical.

We are the only creatures on earth who enjoy sex recreationally. The original function of sex was procreational. From an evolutionary point of view men are still programmed to spread their seed far and wide and women's biological destiny is to reproduce. Social and cultural forces have moved faster than evolutionary development.

■ Anatomy and physiology

In order to help couples improve their sexual relationship the therapist needs to feel comfortable talking about it. Sometimes it is necessary to use the language that clients bring. Sexual vocabulary varies enormously. For example, sexual intercourse may be expressed as:

- sleep with
- go to bed with
- make love
- fuck
- shag
- screw
- bonk
- do it.

The penis may be referred to as:

- willy
- cock
- dick
- prick
- member
- tool
- organ
- rod.

Female genitals may be known as:

- vagina
- vulva
- cunt
- fanny
- hole
- slit
- down there
- front bottom.

The therapist needs to feel at ease with the vocabulary clients use. This enables clients to feel less embarrassed and anxious about sharing their concerns and facilitates a more open communication about a delicate and sensitive problem area in their lives.

■ The genitals

There is a general assumption that because of the amount of detailed information available in the media, clients know what is where, what goes where and what happens next. However, there is a surprising amount of ignorance. The therapist's prime role is to facilitate talking about clients' feelings, but sometimes it is an educational role too. It is important to check clients' levels of knowledge and not to presume that they are well informed.

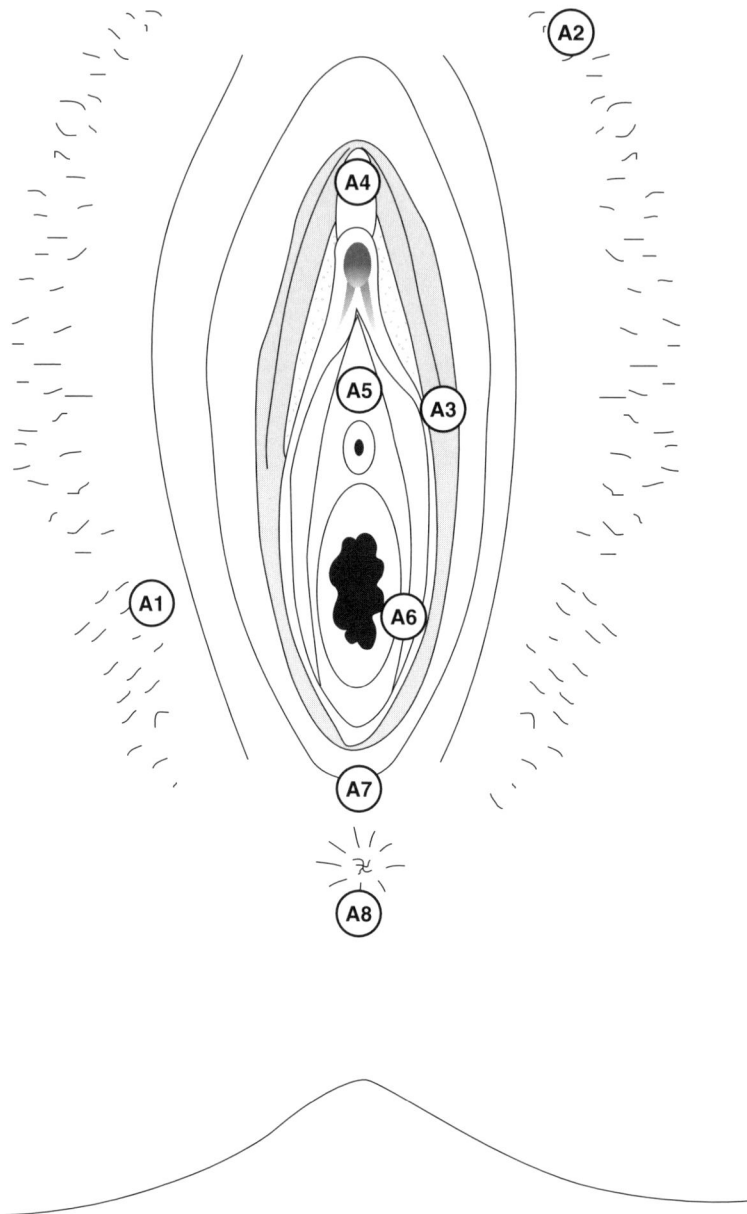

Figure 5.1   Women's genitals: external.

Women: external (Figure 5.1)

The vulva (A1) describes the whole of the external female genitals.

The pubic mound (A2) is the pad of fatty tissue that provides protection for the pubic bone during sex.

The outer and inner labia (A3) are the fleshy lips at the entrance of the vagina. They become engorged with blood and grow bigger during sexual arousal. The inner surfaces of the outer labia have many nerve endings. The inner labia form a protective hood over the clitoris. There is wide variation in size and appearance.

The clitoris (A4). The head of the clitoris can be seen under the clitoral hood.

The urethral opening (A5) is situated just behind the clitoris and carries the urine out of the body.

The hymen (A6) is the membrane that partially covers the entrance to the vagina. It is the traditional sign of virginity, although in many women it is broken by exercise, tampons or masturbation.

The perineum (A7) is the very sensitive area between the back of the vulva and the anus.

The anus (A8) is the opening to the rectum and is also a very sensitive area.

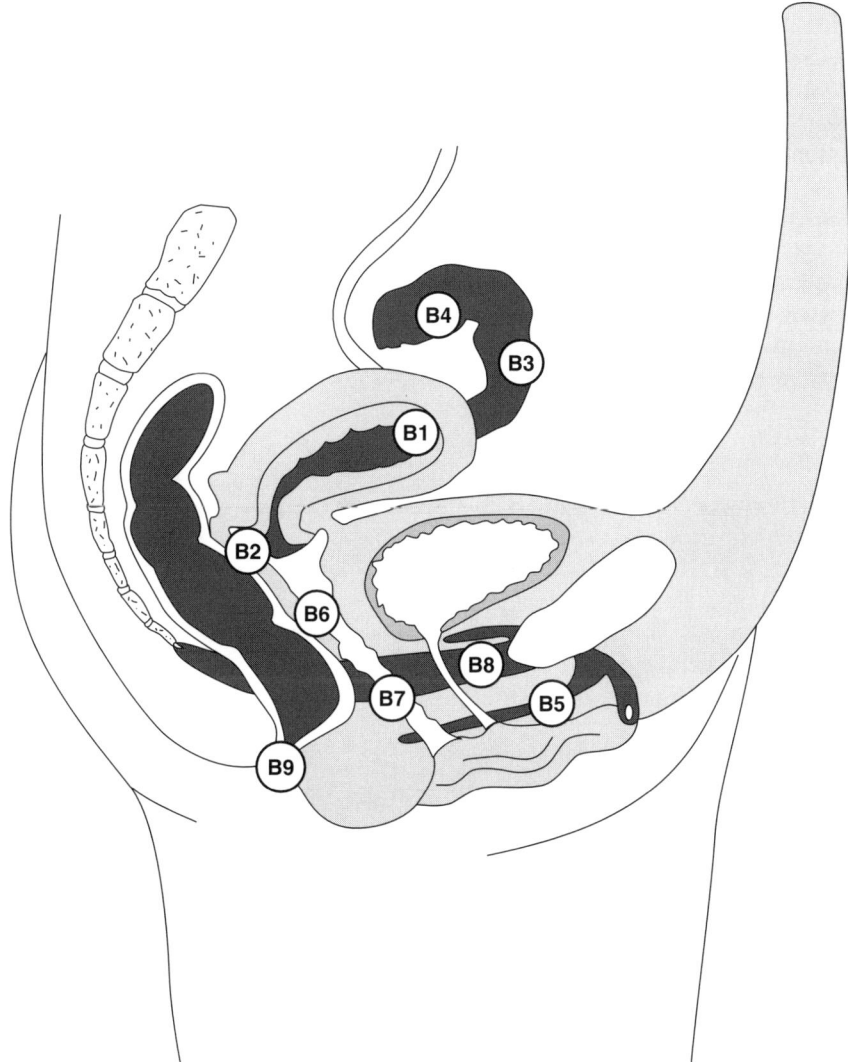

Figure 5.2   Women's genitals: internal.

Women: internal (Figure 5.2)

The uterus (B1) is made up of muscle and other tissues. The lining of the uterus (the endometrium) thickens and is shed every month in menstruation.

The cervix (B2) is the neck of the uterus protruding into the vagina. During orgasm, the cervix dips to help the sperm enter the uterus.

The fallopian tubes (B3) connect to each ovary and carry the egg towards the uterus where it can be fertilised.

The ovaries (B4) store the eggs and produce the hormones oestrogen and progesterone.

The crura (B5) are the internal wing tips of the clitoris situated under the labia.

The vagina (B6) is the passage leading to the cervix and uterus and can expand when necessary.

The G-spot (B7) is the very sensitive tissue around the urethra. Its existence is not certain.

The pubococcygeal muscle (B8). This powerful muscle supports the pelvic floor and contracts during orgasm.

The anal sphincter and the rectum (B9) control the anus and the passage connecting to the colon.

Men: external (Figure 5.3)

The shaft of the penis (C1) is the main part of the penis and contains spongy erectile caverns that fill with blood to produce an erection.

The glans (C2) is the head of the penis and is very sensitive.

The coronal ridge (C3) is the ridge round the base of the glans.

The frenulum (C4) is the triangular fold that goes from the coronal ridge to the glans.

The foreskin (C5) is the roll of skin covering the glans. This is removed in circumcision.

The urethral opening (C6) is the hole at the tip of the penis leading to the urethra through which urine and semen are passed.

The scrotum (C7) is the soft sac hanging below the penis that contains the testicles and monitors their temperature.

The perineum (C8) is the area between the scrotum and the anus, containing a very sensitive central ridge.

The anus (C9) is the opening to the rectum, and is also a very sensitive area.

Men: internal (Figure 5.4)

The testicles (D1), or testes, produce the sperm. The left testicle is lower than the right one because the tubes it contains are longer.

The epididymis (D2) connects each testicle to the vas deferens and transports the sperm.

The vas deferens (D3) connects the epididymis to the seminal vesicles. They are the ejaculatory ducts that are cut in a vasectomy.

The seminal vesicles (D4) secrete seminal fluid and contract to pass the fluid into the ejaculatory ducts.

The corpora cavernosa (D5) is the spongy erectile tissue that fills with blood to produce an erection.

The urethral sphincter muscles and the urethra (D6). The sphincter muscles contract to allow either urine or sperm to be expelled via the urethra.

Cowper's glands (D7) secrete the pre-seminal fluid that precedes orgasm.

The prostate gland (D8) secretes some of the fluid that makes up the ejaculation and pushes it through the urethra.

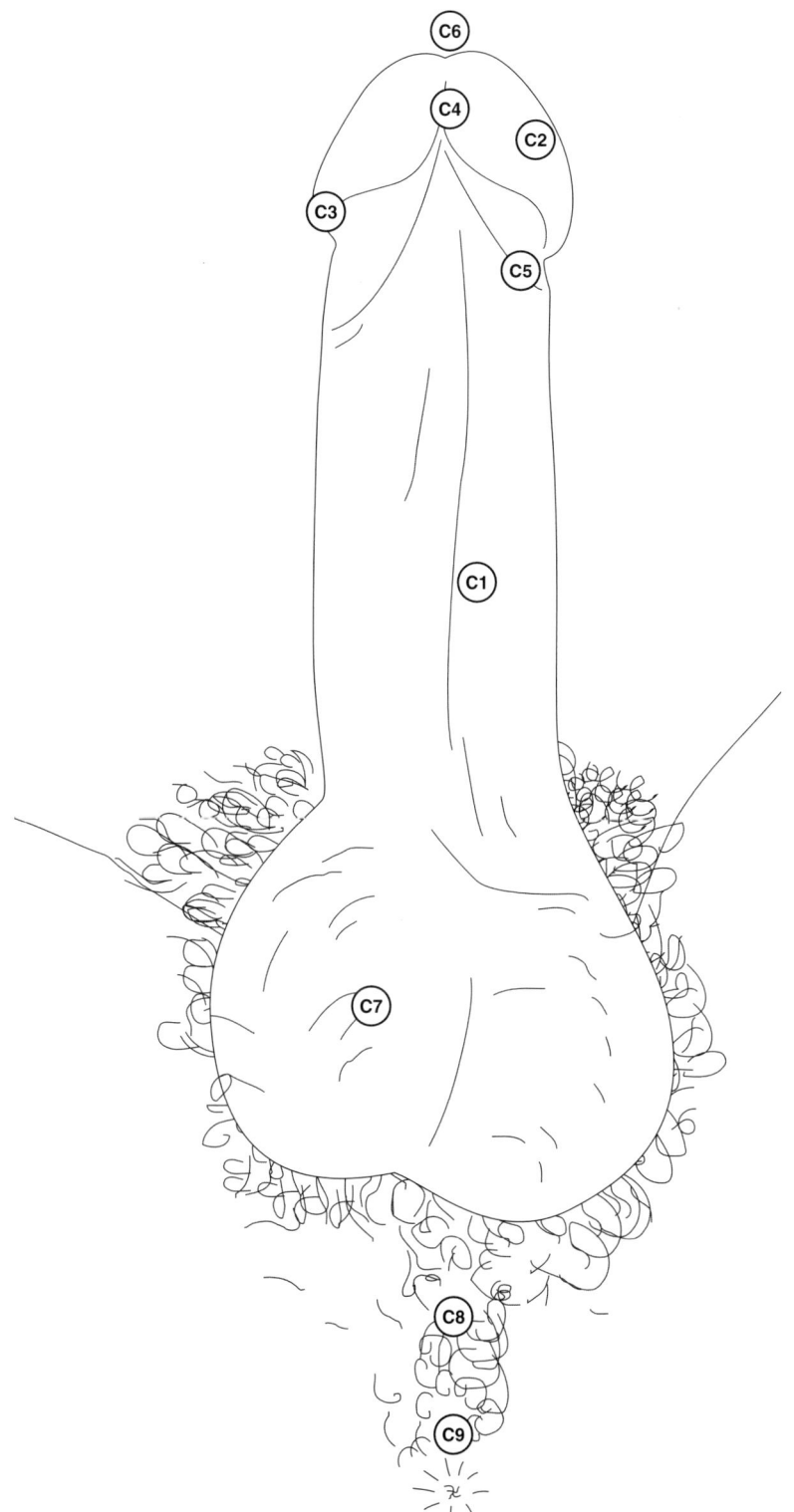

Figure 5.3 Men's genitals: external.

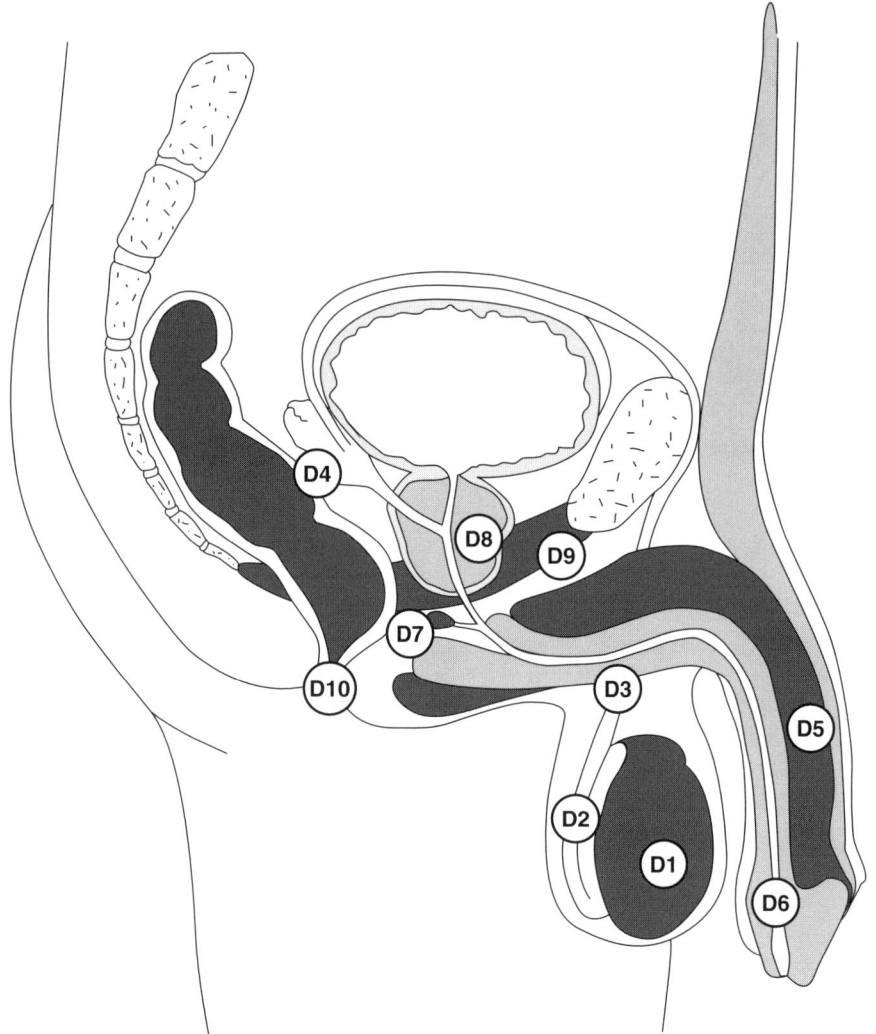

Figure 5.4   Men's genitals: internal.

The pubococcygeal muscle (D9) is a powerful muscle that supports the pelvic floor and contracts during orgasm.

The anal sphincter and the rectum (D10) control the anus and the passage connecting to the colon.

■ The phases of sexual response

Desire is a subtle and complex mechanism controlled by the brain, the senses, the environment and the quality of the relationship. It is a phenomenon that is:

- physiological
- neurological

- hormonal
- psychological
- emotional
- mental.

Arousal is affected by thoughts, feelings and fantasies and can best be seen as a circuit (*see* Figure 5.5).

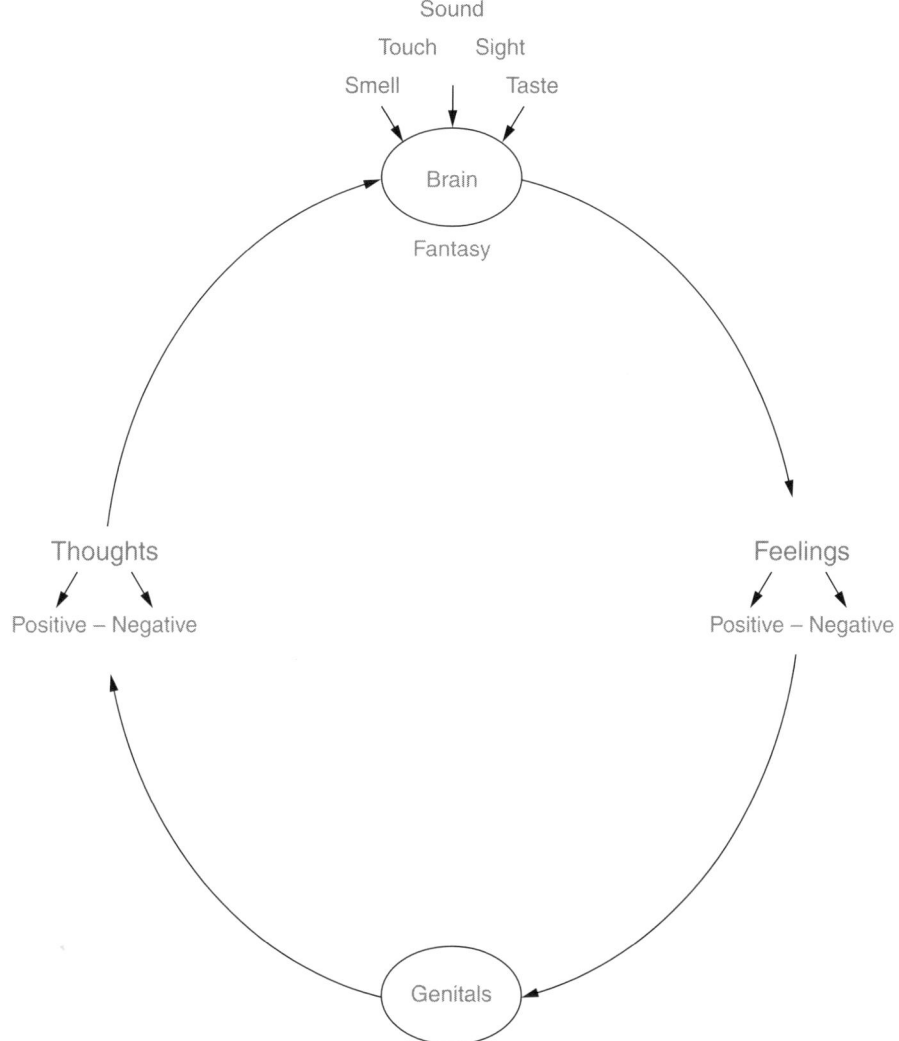

Figure 5.5 The arousal circuit.

The arousal circuit can be broken at any point. Couples need to be able to communicate with each other about what turns them on and off, what engages and disengages their brains.

The therapist can use the arousal circuit with clients as a diagnostic and therapeutic tool. The arousal circuit:

- explains the process of desire
- identifies what helps and what hinders, what gets it going and what shuts it down
- gives insight into break points
- distinguishes between conscious and unconscious thoughts
- facilitates changes in thoughts and behaviour.

The stages of sexual response are:

- excitement
- arousal
- plateau
- pre-orgasm
- orgasm
- resolution.

This can be expressed as the ladder of desire (*see* Figure 5.6).

Men and women will have different experiences and expectations of how they go up and down the ladder during sex and will usually function at different speeds and in different time frames.

■ Ground level to excitement

Women: This is about mood, feelings and engaging the senses.
Men: This is a far less important stage for men. The urge to move on up the ladder is strong.

■ Arousal

Women: This is where physical changes start to occur. Stimulation causes vaginal lubrication, swelling of the clitoris, thickening of the labia, nipple erection and quickening pulse.
Men: This step is faster in men. Increased blood flow brings the erection. The scrotum and testicles elevate, the nipples increase in sensitivity, and the pulse quickens.

■ Plateau

Women: The clitoris retracts into the clitoral hood and is now hypersensitive. The labia and vagina swell, the uterus and cervix elevate, the breasts enlarge, a flush may occur over the chest, neck and face, respiration and pulse increase in rate.
Men: The erection is maintained, the testicles enlarge and elevate, respiration and pulse increase in rate.

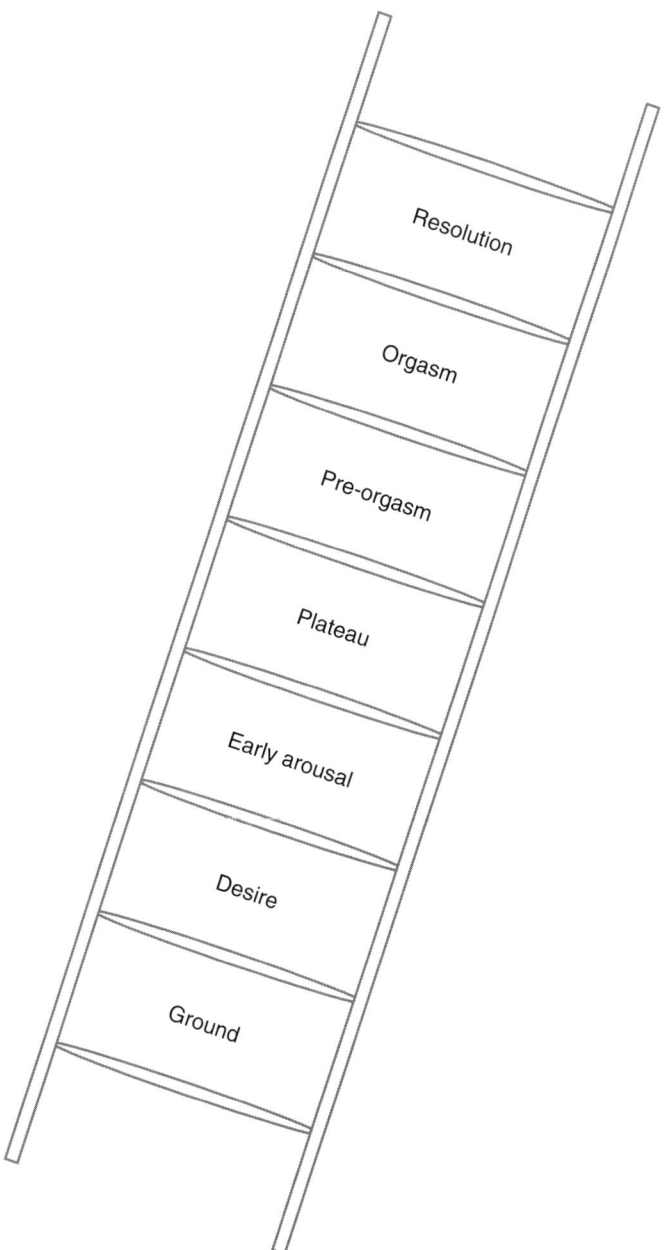

Figure 5.6   The ladder of desire.

■ Pre-orgasm

Women: The time needed to move from plateau to pre-orgasm varies considerably and may not occur at all. When it does occur, the point of orgasmic inevitability is reached.

Men: The prostate contracts, bringing ejaculatory inevitability.

■ Orgasm

Women: This is a series of 5–15 contractions every 0.8 seconds which can be felt as anything from a clitoral or vaginal fluttering to powerful uterine contractions. Respiration and pulse will reach their maximum rate.
Men: The seminal vesicles, vas deferens and urethra contract, causing the emission of seminal fluid – the ejaculation. Respiration and pulse will reach their maximum rate.

■ Resolution (after-glow)

Women: Everything returns to normal, the cervix dips down into the vagina. There is a feeling of well-being and relaxation. Women who experience multiple orgasms will return several times to the plateau, pre-orgasm and orgasm phases.
Men: The penis detumesces, the testicles return to their normal size, the body relaxes, often to the point of sleepiness.

The refractory period (the time needed before erection and orgasm can be reached again) varies from a few minutes in adolescence to several hours in older men.

Understanding what happens during sex and being able to talk about it will bring great improvements to a couple's sexual relationship. It is particularly helpful to know that men and women move at different speeds up and down the ladder of desire so that each one can adjust their expectations and actions accordingly.

■ Problems that can affect good sex

Good sex may be adversely affected by many physical events. These are now described.

■ Illness

In women
- Miscarriages, abortion, childbirth, episiotomy, uterine prolapse.
- PMT, endometriosis, menopause, hormonal imbalance.
- Polycystic ovaries, blocked fallopian tubes, fibroids.
- Cancer of the cervix, ovaries, uterus, breasts.
- Haemorrhoids, cystitis, stress incontinence.
- Thrush, vaginitis, pelvic inflammatory disease.

In men
- Undescended testicles.
- Foreskin problems.
- Orchitis.
- Prostate problems, cancer.
- Urinary infections.
- Hormone problems.

In both
Sexually transmitted diseases including:

- herpes
- genital warts
- chlamydia
- fungal infections
- gonorrhoea
- syphilis
- HIV/AIDS.

Other conditions:

- cancer, multiple sclerosis, diabetes, cardiovascular problems, arthritis, back pain, ME
- depression, anxiety, stress, exhaustion, mental illness
- injury, accidents, trauma, surgery, pain
- abuse of drugs, alcohol, cigarettes.

■ Medication

- Blood pressure lowering drugs, cholesterol lowering drugs.
- Anti-depressants, tranquillisers, anti-psychotics, neuroleptics.
- Corticosteroids, contraceptive pill, hormone replacement therapy (HRT), other hormone treatments.

Any of these prescribed medications may affect sexual response and performance.

■ Contraception

All forms of birth control may affect sexual response and performance:

- condom
- Pill
- IUD
- implant
- diaphragm
- morning-after pill
- withdrawal
- rhythm method
- termination
- vasectomy
- sterilisation.

■ Infertility

The treatments and processes currently available are increasingly complex. Issues that may have a negative impact on a couple's sexual relationship include:

- sex on demand
- procreation not recreation
- loss of intimacy
- medicalisation
- hormone disturbance
- minor surgery
- miscarriages
- mood swings
- disappointment
- sense of failure
- loss of self-esteem
- loss
- grief
- anxiety
- depression
- stress
- guilt
- blame
- shame
- anger
- despair
- obsession
- breakdown of relationship.

Couples may not experience all of these events and feelings, but the therapist needs to be aware of these possibilities and be able to raise and discuss them.

■ Singular sex: sex for one

One can assume that most men masturbate but it is surprising to discover that many women do not.

It can be useful in therapy to find out why. A woman's attitude to masturbation reflects her feelings about herself, her body and her sexual responses. Just talking about it in a safe place will be extremely helpful and liberating. It will also be permission-giving. The most useful aid to masturbation is the simple vibrator (not to be confused with the dildo, an artificial penis). Applied externally in the clitoral area, one is virtually guaranteed to reach orgasm.

For women and men who do not really know their bodies and need guidance, there is a series of exercises to be carried out at leisure and in comfort at home. These are known as self-focus and they are more sensual than sexual to start with. They were pioneered by the sex therapists Masters and Johnson in the United States in 1966. The therapist needs to introduce these exercises with sensitivity and make sure that the client has fully understood the instructions.

■ Self-focus for women

Exercise 1 for women

This exercise will help you to get more acquainted with your body. You may also learn new things about how your body looks and how subtly it works; new things about how your body feels when it is touched, especially in places you hadn't thought of before. When you feel familiar with your body you will be more able to share what feels good.

Set aside approximately 30 minutes when you have undisturbed privacy. For this exercise you will need, if possible, a full-length mirror, a hand mirror and a warm room. Try to clear your mind of worries and responsibilities in order to focus on what you are doing.

Now take a warm bath or shower but not just to get clean. If bathing, experience it in a new way. You may like to use some bath salts, oil or foam. Use this time as an opportunity to become aware of the feel of the warm water and the different parts of your body. Lower yourself slowly into the bath and concentrate on how the different parts of you react to the wetness and the warmth. For example, it may feel quite different to the legs than to the small of the back. If showering, turn around under the shower, letting the water hit different parts of your body. Experiment with different water pressures. How does it feel as the water strikes your shoulders, stomach and arms? Now soap yourself, using hands or a flannel. Try both. Be aware of different textures on your skin. Are there other ways of feeling good? Do some areas feel good in a soothing sort of way, while others are invigorating? Be aware as well of the sound of the water.

When you have finished your bath or shower, get dried using a warm towel. Really concentrate on how it feels to dry yourself. Try patting gently then rubbing hard. Which does your skin prefer? Let yourself really experience the drying process. Don't rush through it. Out of habit we often focus on just the main parts. Spend time on the other parts, such as ears, hands, fingers, toes.

Now stand in front of the mirror and notice the overall shape of your body. Pay attention to what you are doing. It may not be easy at first. Your mind may wander. If this happens simply bring your mind back to this task. Study your body. Try to look at it from all angles, using a hand mirror to get a good view of your back. While your face will be very familiar to you, your body may be less so. Notice its asymmetry (the difference between the right-hand side and the left-hand side). Notice what hair distribution there may be; this varies from person to person. We all have some on our bodies. Sometimes there is hair surrounding the areola (the dark area around the nipple). It can also extend up from the genital area to the navel or it can extend down the thighs.

How do you feel about this? Women are often inhibited about their body because of scars or stretch marks. Stretch marks are very common and often occur around the hips, stomach and legs, whether you have had children or not.

Most people start off by noticing what they don't like about their body – breasts too big or too small and so on. We often pick up media ideas on how we ought to look, but styles, shape and fashions change and are we really being realistic?

If, however, you feel you are seriously underweight or overweight you may be prompted to do something about this. Bear in mind that we often cannot change the way we are.

When you have spent enough time looking at yourself, wrap up warmly and relax or get dressed leisurely.

What have you learned from this exercise? What have you noticed or discovered about your body that you didn't know before?

You need to repeat this exercise several times before you become familiar with the way you look.

Exercise 2 for women

Start with a relaxing bath or shower, and while drying yourself remind yourself of the things you have learned in Exercise 1. In Exercise 2 you are going to extend your physical exploration.

Use the sensitivity of your hands to notice and appreciate the varying textures of your body. Start from your head and slowly work your way downwards. Be aware, almost as if you are touching your body for the first time. Look at and touch the front of your body, noticing the feel of your skin. Explore your hands, arms, shoulders and breasts. Move slowly over the stomach, let your fingers run through your pubic hair, inside your thighs, legs, feet and toes. Relax as you do this and value your body even if you are not what you consider to be an ideal shape. Become aware of the different shapes and textures and be aware of how each part feels. Which parts do you enjoy touching and what sort of touch do they most respond to? Concentrate on what you are doing and try not to let your mind wander. If it does, simply bring it back to the task.

The first time you do this exercise it may feel rather strange and uncomfortable. For many of us there are long-established taboos about touching the body and especially noticing sensations of pleasure and arousal. After a second or third time you can let your hands explore further over your breasts as you fondle them. You may notice your breasts and nipple size change as you fondle them. Your breasts become firmer and your nipples may become erect. Run your hands over your pubic hair again and over your genitals and become aware of their shape, texture and temperature.

Sometimes use a dry hand and other times use oil, lotion or talcum powder to enjoy the different sensations and responses of your body.

As in Exercise 1, when you have finished wrap up warmly and relax or get dressed slowly.

What have you learned from this exercise and what have you noticed or discovered about your body that you didn't know before? Repeat this exercise several times.

Exercise 3 for women

This exercise is intended to encourage you to experiment and explore further physically and sensually and to learn more about what, where and how you enjoy being touched. For this you will need a fairly large hand mirror.

Always start with a relaxing bath or shower. Work through the first two stages. This will help to relax you and will reinforce the bits you feel comfortable with. Now prop yourself up against something firm like a headboard or pillows. Bend your knees and open your legs to expose your genitals. Position and prop up the hand mirror so that your hands are free and you can see your genitals.

Start by looking at and touching your pubic hair. Note again how it is distributed, where it starts and ends, also its texture. This hair is necessary because it protects this very sensitive part of your body from irritation and perspiration. Now move onto your genital lips or labia. The outer lips are also covered by pubic hair for protection. Identify the outer and inner lips, the inner being smaller than the outer ones. You will need to use your fingers to pull the lips apart to see them properly. No two women are alike and the variation in size and shape differs vastly from woman to woman. Sometimes the inner lips are more prominent and hang down between the outer lips. The colour of the lips also varies. So, note your size and colour. Feel the lips and notice the difference in their texture and temperature.

You will have to pull open the lips fairly wide apart to expose your vagina, the urethra and the clitoris. The inner lips usually meet at the top of the clitoral hood, the bit that protects the clitoris. The urethra is between the vagina and the clitoris. When you have found them look for the anus and perineum – the muscle between the vagina and the anus. Often the clitoris, which is a woman's most sensitive part, is difficult to find as it is protected by the clitoral hood and in an unaroused state it may be withdrawn and difficult to locate. There are considerable variations in the size of the clitoris.

Now let your fingers explore and feel around the mouth of the vagina. Do this stage slowly. Initially just feel around the lips, the clitoris and the vagina. When you feel OK let your fingers explore further and feel inside your vagina. Try to identify the ridges on the inner walls. Note the texture changes as you feel further inside. The vagina is usually moist. Occasionally dryness can occur. You may like to use a lotion or lubricating gel to do this exercise.

You may become aroused during this exercise and that is OK. You will be able to notice how the clitoris becomes hard and erect, how the labia change colour and the vagina becomes moist.

When you have finished this exercise take time, relax and think about it all, especially the new things you have learned and what you can share with your partner. As before, it is useful to repeat this exercise several times.

■ Self-focus for men

Exercise 1 for men

This exercise will help you to get more acquainted with your body. You may also learn new things about how your body looks and how subtly it works; new things about how your body feels when it is touched, especially in places you hadn't thought of before. When you feel familiar with your body you will be more able to share what feels good.

Set aside approximately 30 minutes when you have undisturbed privacy. For this exercise you will need, if possible, a full-length mirror, a hand mirror and a warm room. Try to clear your mind of worries and responsibilities in order to focus on what you are doing.

Now take a warm bath or shower but not just to get clean. If bathing, experience it in a new way. You may like to use some bath salts, oil or foam. Use this time as an opportunity to become aware of the feel of the warm water and the different parts of your body. Lower yourself slowly into the bath and concentrate on how the different parts of you react to the wetness and the warmth. For example, it may feel quite different to the legs than to the small of the back. If showering, turn around under the shower, letting the water hit different parts of your body. Experiment with different water pressures. How does it feel as the water strikes your shoulders, stomach and arms? Now soap yourself, using hands or a flannel. Try both. Be aware of different textures on your skin. Are there other ways of feeling good? Do some areas feel good in a soothing sort of way, while others are invigorating? Be aware as well of the sound of the water.

When you have finished your bath or shower, get dried using a warm towel. Really concentrate on how it feels to dry yourself. Try patting gently then rubbing hard. Which does your skin prefer? Let yourself really experience the drying process. Don't rush through it (out of habit we often focus on just the main parts). Spend time on the other parts such as ears, hands, fingers, toes.

Now stand in front of the mirror and notice the overall shape of your body. Pay attention to what you are doing. It may not be easy at first. Your mind may wander. If this happens simply bring your mind back to this task. Study your body. Try to look at it from all angles, using a hand mirror to get a good view of your back. While your face will be very familiar to you, your body may be less so. Notice its asymmetry (the difference between the right-hand side and the left-hand side). Notice what hair distribution there may be. Is it restricted to the protected area of under arms and lower pelvis or does it extend to other areas? How do you feel about this?

Notice the muscle distribution and whether or not it is covered by fatty tissue, either all over or in specific areas. Perhaps ask yourself why you may be more covered in some areas than others, or why more muscular. How do you feel about those areas?

Let your eyes travel down your body looking at each part in turn. Look down your chest to your hips, your penis and your scrotum. View yourself from different angles perhaps using a hand mirror. Some men can be secretly sensitive about the size, shape and colour of their penis. In fact every man sees his penis in a foreshortened way as he looks down on it – while, when he glances at another man's penis, say in a changing room, he views it from the side. Actually, in an erect state, there is not a great deal of variation in size.

Ask yourself, how do you feel about what you see? How do these things make you feel about yourself sexually? Where do your ideas of how a man should look come from? Like most of us you may have got them from the media. Is this realistic? Is it important anyway?

When you have spent enough time looking at yourself, wrap up warmly and relax or get dressed slowly.

What have you learned from this exercise? What have you noticed or discovered about your body that you didn't know before?

You need to repeat this exercise several times before you become familiar with the way you look.

Exercise 2 for men

Start with a relaxing bath or shower, and while drying remind yourself of the things you have learned in Exercise 1 when you used your visual senses. In this exercise you are going to extend your investigation into physical exploration.

Use the sensitivity of your hands to notice and appreciate the varying textures of your body. Start from the feet and slowly work your way upwards. Be aware, almost as if you are seeing your body for the first time. Look at and touch the front of your body, noticing the feel of your chest, your breast area and nipples. How responsive are those areas to touch? Relax as you do this and value your body even if you are not what you consider to be an ideal shape.

Concentrate on what you are doing and try not to let your mind wander. If it does, simply bring it back to the task. Now start to move your hands slowly downwards and feel the gradual change from a flattish pelvis to the penis. Notice how your pubic hair feels under your fingers. If this produces any feelings of arousal and/or discomfort try to understand why those feelings have come about. For many people there are long-established taboos about touching and noticing sensations in the genital area, other than in washing and toilet functions.

Run your fingers over your pelvis and scrotum. Notice the varying textures – the smooth glans head and contrasting feeling of scrotum and foreskin. If your penis is soft, notice its weight in your hand, the texture of the skin, and extend this to an examination of the scrotum. Use not only the palm and fingers for touching but the back of the hand as well. This exercise is not intended to produce arousal or erection but sometimes it can. Whatever happens is fine. If aroused, notice how the penis takes up its own weight and also notice any tightening of the scrotum. Use a hand mirror to see the underside of the penis and scrotum – your partner may be more familiar with this view than you are. See how everything fits together. Identify the perineum, the area between scrotum and anus.

Exercise 3 for men

This exercise is intended to encourage you to explore and experiment further, physically and sensually, and to learn more about where and how you enjoy being touched.

Always start with a relaxing bath or shower. While doing so recall what you have already learned.

Explore your genitals with your finger. If you press in above your penis you can feel your pubic bone. Now gently squeeze the scrotum above the testicles with one finger in front and one behind the scrotal sack. You will be able to feel the vas deferens. This connects the testes to the base of the bladder and feels like a cord. Now gently stroke your penis, scrotum and the area behind the scrotum, paying close attention to the various sensations produced. Try different types of touching. Note which areas are more sensitive and which areas are less sensitive. Take your time and learn as much as you can.

If you become aroused, take this opportunity to notice the changes that have taken place. Arousal often increases body temperature and flushing can take place on the chest and neck. Your scrotum will probably darken in colour and its skin will thicken. The testicles will rise up and move closer to the body. Your penis may also darken in colour and the veins will become more prominent as it becomes engorged. The colour changes are often only obvious on fair skin. If you press a finger between your scrotum you will be able to feel the bulb of your penis that is back inside your body. If you did have an erection take note of what touches or sensations produced it.

When you have finished this exercise take time, relax and think about it all, especially the new things you have learned and what you can share with your partner.

■ Kegel exercises

Kegel exercises are used to strengthen the pubococcygeal (PC, pelvic floor) muscles. This is a group of muscles which encircle the vagina and urethra in women and the base of the penis and urethra in men.

1 To locate the muscles, urinate with your legs apart and stop the flow of urine mid-stream several times. It is the PC muscles you are using to do this. Once you have located these muscles do not use the exercise in future when urinating as this may not allow the bladder to empty completely and may lead to infection. It is purely an exercise to help you locate the muscles.
2 Tighten the muscles for three seconds and then relax them for a count of three and then tighten again. At first you may not be able to hold the tension for a whole three seconds, but you will develop the ability when the muscles grow stronger. NB: You should not feel your tummy muscles tighten at the same time.
3 Now tighten and relax the muscles ten times as quickly as you can so that they seem to 'flutter'. You will probably need to practise for a while before you will be able to control the muscles in this way.

4 The final step is to bear down, pushing through the vagina or pelvis rather than the anus. Hold that tension for three seconds.
5 Try to do this set of exercises ten times – twice a day, if you can – for a week. Then at least once a day thereafter.

These exercises are intended to increase your awareness of the sensations these muscles can produce. They will help to intensify sensations of intercourse for both you and your partner. This is because the PC muscles are among those that contract during orgasm. Kegel exercises are helpful too after childbirth and for most post-menopausal women because, by increasing the blood flow to the vaginal area, they help to maintain vaginal lubrication. They are also extremely helpful for men with premature ejaculation as they strengthen and help awareness of the point of ejaculatory inevitability. The exercises are also a help in counteracting stress incontinence.

■ Fantasies and variations
■ Sexual fantasies

Given that the brain is where sexual arousal starts, the use of fantasy is extremely effective. As with masturbation, there is a marked gender difference in the use of fantasy. It comes naturally to men but some women seem to need encouragement or permission to allow their minds to wander along the paths of sexual fantasy. For those whose imaginations need stimulating there is a vast body of erotic literature available without the need to resort to pornography.

Many couples are happy to share their fantasies and enhance their sexual experiences. For clients who are cautious about exploring their sexual fantasies, the therapist may ask them each to write down a fantasy and read it out to each other. This would take place outside the therapy. It is useful to remind them that fantasies do not have to be acted out. This exercise is very helpful in increasing one's awareness about oneself and one's partner as sexual beings. The relationship will invariably be enriched.

■ Sexual variations

Genital intercourse is not the only way to have good sex. Most of the body's orifices are highly sensitive with many nerve endings. Both the giving and receiving of oral and anal sex can be immensely pleasurable.

Some couples enjoy using sex toys, role-play, dressing up, the use of rubber or leather, bondage or domination. Some will indulge in telephone sex or even sex in public places. As long as there is genuine mutual consent and no unwanted manipulation or exploitation, anything that is agreed can contribute to good sex.

Most of us have access to the Internet, videos, books, magazines, sex shops, chat-lines and personal ads. All kinds of pornography are easily available. As therapists we need to know what is acceptable to us without being judgemental to our clients. If we are not comfortable talking about these issues, our clients will not be either.

It is of course essential to maintain firm boundaries and not allow feelings such as disapproval, distaste, curiosity or arousal to influence the therapy.

■ Cultural and religious expectations

In the world's major religions good sex is as much about giving pleasure as getting it within the context of a spiritual union. Although most of the world's societies are patriarchal, women are in general honoured within the framework of marriage.

It is worth noting that in western societies sexuality is out there, in fashion, journalism, TV, cinema, the Internet, etc. Yet Christianity brings with it a legacy of guilt and shame, repression and inhibition with the concept of sin and repentance. There is often a prurient interest in the forbidden and a puritanical reaction to genuine eroticism. Other religions reject western cultural decadence and insist on privacy and modesty. However, a woman's sexuality is much valued within the confines of marriage and her pleasure is an important part of the relationship.

Muslim women may wear the veil, the chador or the burqa to protect them from the unwanted gaze of men, but in private their bodies are often finely dressed and bejewelled. Sex within marriage is part of providing love, joy and companionship with total commitment.

The Perfumed Garden, an erotic how-to book from ancient Persia, is about mutual pleasure and inventiveness in sexual practices.

Hinduism is renowned for the *Kama Sutra*, erotic carvings and miniatures, and Tantric sex, which brings a spiritual value to sex.

Kissing is as far as it goes in Bollywood movies, but the practice of sex behind closed doors is very different.

Buddhism also includes Tantric sex, which is about the release of energy and reaching spiritual union and enlightenment. Figures of sexual union symbolise the fusion of compassion and wisdom.

The Japanese and Chinese have a fine tradition of erotic art. *The Pillow Book* is their ancient sex manual.

In Judaism it is part of the marriage contract that the husband gives the wife regular sex and ensures that sex is pleasurable for her. The sexual relationship requires commitment and responsibility. The Hebrew word for sex comes from the same root as the word meaning 'to know', as used in the Bible. This illustrates the intimacy of heart, mind and body that is shared between a loving couple. The Song of Solomon in the Old Testament is one of the most poetic pieces of erotic writing.

It is important in couples therapy to be aware of these cultural and religious values and beliefs because we need to know what our clients' expectations are. When working with bi-cultural couples this becomes even more important. Currently there is a dearth of ethnic minority counsellors and a growing need in the community.

Sometimes our own assumptions may distract us. The therapist may need to acknowledge difference, not just between the couple, but between the couple and herself. When we are ignorant about cultural practices we need to ask the clients for information. It is important never to presume anything.

■ Sex and the life cycle

The nature of good sex will change throughout the life cycle and will reflect the physical and emotional changes that men and women go through as they negotiate each stage.

■ Psychosexual development

- *Birth to 18 months: ORAL.* The developments during this stage will have a profound influence on the person's sexuality in adulthood. These include attachment, touch, holding and caressing, merging and separating, gratification, mirroring, play, tolerance of frustration, and good-enough meeting of needs.
- *18 months to 3: ANAL.* The issues here are around power and control, punishment and praise, order and discipline; also awareness of the body and body functions, the discovery and naming of genitals. This is simpler for boys because their genitals are visible and harder for girls whose genitals are mainly hidden. This is also the stage where one may have to deal with guilt, shame, embarrassment and inhibition, all of which may manifest in adult sexuality.
- *3 to 5: GENITAL/OEDIPAL.* Gender identity is developed here through identification with the same-sex parent. Feelings of ambivalence, anxiety, rivalry, envy and jealousy all need to be negotiated. There is loss of sole claim to the mother, exclusion from the parents' sexual relationship, and perhaps the arrival of a sibling and the subsequent displacement within the family.
- *5 to 12: LATENCY.* This is a time of curiosity, information-gathering and learning about sexual matters. The child is not yet physically able to have sex but will be interested in exploring genitals, particularly with an opposite-sex friend.
- *12 to 20: ADOLESCENCE.* Puberty brings body changes, menstruation, wet dreams, sexualisation, and issues around body image. Fantasies and masturbation will increase. There will be sexual experimentation, experiential learning and acting out, group identification, and separation from the family. This is a sexually very intense stage.
- *20 to 40: ADULTHOOD.* This is the time of serial relationships, falling in love, bonding and commitment. The purpose and meaning of sex will change and transform from 'in love' to 'loving', especially through pregnancies and babies. Couples may unconsciously identify with the developmental stage of their infants. Life events such as career changes, illness, family problems and financial hardship will bring stresses that may adversely affect the sexual relationship.
- *40 to 70: MATURITY.* This is a time when mid-life crises coincide with the menopause, adolescent children and ageing parents. One's sexuality may decrease as it is affected by ageing and health problems just as one's children's sexual activities are rapidly increasing. The sexual relationship will require time and attention if it is to remain satisfactory and fulfilling.
- *70 to ?: OLD AGE.* The task in old age is to do with loss and letting go. Physical problems may increase with physiological changes. These include a decrease in libido and in erectile ability, and atrophy and loss of lubrication in women. However, the pioneer post-war generation is breaking new ground in terms of their sexuality. Women on HRT are remaining vigorous and energetic and men are still able to perform thanks to Viagra and similar drugs. Divorce and widowhood no longer mean the end of one's sex life.

Example: 'Useless prick'

Jack and Ellie came to therapy because Jack had developed erectile problems, which seemed rooted in developmental difficulties. Jack had erections on waking and had no problem masturbating, but he was a failure with Ellie, and felt blamed and ashamed. (*See* Figure 5.7.)

Jack had been attracted to Ellie, who was very beautiful, because he thought she was warm and loving and would give him the intimacy and affection that he was lacking from his mother. This was a projective idealised fantasy. Ellie turned out to be as hostile and rejecting as his mother.

Jack was a disappointment to his mother because she had very much wanted a daughter. Her feelings for him had been ambivalent from the start. When his younger brother was born, she had no time for him and he was sent straight to nursery school. As the middle child, Jack was more or less left to get on with life on his own. He did not get much attention from either parent. His mother left when he was 18, and he left home for university. Her parting words to her husband were that he was a 'useless prick'.

Ellie's mother was demanding and manipulative. She and Jack had strong, difficult mothers and emasculated fathers in common. Ellie was close to her father, but irritated by his passivity with her mother. He adored Ellie and spoilt her but could not stand up for himself. (Jack's penis could not stand up for itself.) She did not understand why he had not left her mother. Both Jack and Ellie were repeating their parents' marriages.

In therapy, Jack was able to recognise the recurring patterns, but Ellie became more hostile and defensive. Just as his mother had castrated his father, so Ellie had castrated him and shamed him with his inadequacy. He had identified with his father, the 'useless prick'.

Eventually Jack realised that he would have to end the relationship because Ellie was not prepared to own anything or make any changes. She could not admit how disappointed she was with her father's weakness, nor could she let go of her narcissistic fantasy of being extra-special to him. She was frustrated because Jack had also failed to make her feel extra-special. She blamed his erectile problems, but would not admit that she was a part of the problem.

Both Jack and Ellie were acting out in the relationship their unsatisfactory Oedipal issues. Ellie withdrew from the therapy and the relationship came to an end. This was a repeat of his mother leaving his father and their marriage coming to an end.

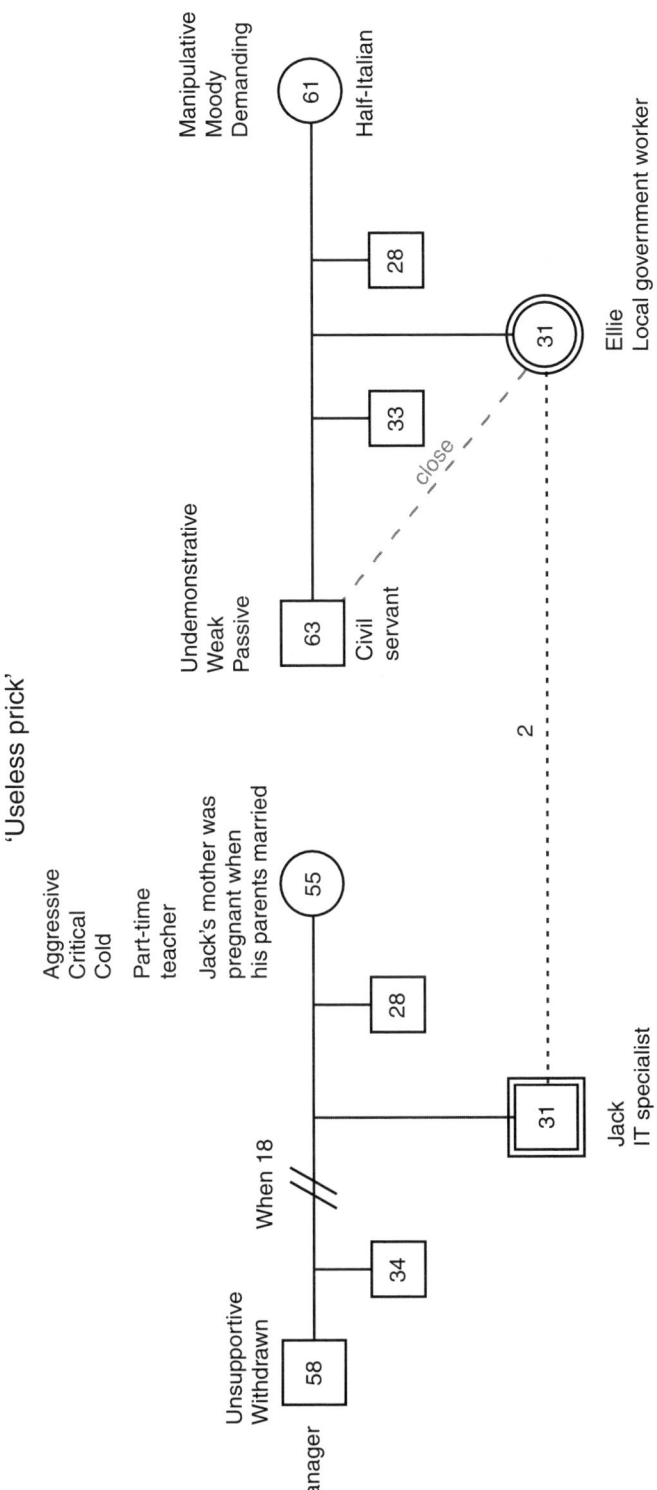

Figure 5.7 'Useless prick.'

CHAPTER 6

Bad sex

Bad sex includes behaviour that is driven by compulsion and the need for power and control. It can be violent and debasing, sordid and shameful, bizarre and risky. Chosen objects, i.e. fetishistic objects, and situations that are compulsively repeated take on a particular sexual meaning. There is often a lack of mutual consent, an imposed secrecy. Hatred is eroticised; boundaries are broken.

Bad sex usually comes with a history of early deprivation and frustration, a desperate and narcissistic need for satisfaction or even punishment, expressed in the acting out of taboo desires and fantasies.

'Sad' sex is another form of bad sex, when sex between a couple becomes dutiful and boring, or is affected by repression, inhibition or ignorance.

Is anonymous sex – often illicit, with no degree of intimacy but some degree of thrill – bad sex? Men – and it is almost always male behaviour – who frequent prostitutes, massage parlours or lap-dancing clubs, or indulge in kerb crawling, voyeurism or exhibitionism, are usually unable to sustain a lasting and profound sexual relationship. The repetition of bad sex in situations they can control, either with force or by payment, brings temporary respite to their frustrated desires.

With the advent of Internet porn and swap clubs, sexual behaviour is breaching new frontiers in the search for increasing novelty and stimulation. Anything is permitted. Children are becoming sexualised at an even earlier age. Sex is marketed as an activity where instant gratification is encouraged and expected.

The emotional and psychological fall-out of bad sex is considerable, not just for the victim but also for the instigator. As a client group they both need sensitive work with an experienced and confident therapist, who will maintain firm boundaries.

■ Sexual abuse
■ Definition

Sexual abuse may be:

- visual, as in exhibitionism
- verbal, in the use of inappropriate sexual language or threats
- physical, when touch is sexualised.

It may be oral or anal, masturbatory or penetrative.

It is often violent, as in sexual assault and rape, and always manipulative and exploitative.

Lack of consent and imbalance of power are major features.

It occurs between males and females, males and males, and more rarely the instigator may be a female abusing a male or a female.

The victims are usually pre-pubescent or developmentally immature.

■ Splits

Victims of sexual abuse experience major splits. Some of these splits that are reflected in the family and wider community include:

• belief	• disbelief
• reality	• fantasy
• love	• hate
• omnipotence	• powerlessness
• good guy	• bad guy
• body	• head
• physical sensation	• emotional response
• special	• defiled.

The people who are involved in sexual abuse frequently become polarised:

• children	• parents
• mothers	• fathers
• families	• relatives
• therapists	• lawyers
• social workers	• psychiatrists
• nurses	• doctors
• mass audience	• mass media.

The major emotional states that the victim may feel reflect the split between positive and negative and include the following.

Negative	*Positive*
Shame	Love
Guilt	Pleasure
Disgust	Desire
Self-hatred	Attachment
Confusion	Affection
Anger	Intimacy
Fear	Loyalty
Dependency	Feeling special
Loss of boundary	Sharing a secret
Loss of safety	Power
Loss of security	
Loss of trust	
Isolation	
Abandonment	
Betrayal	
Retribution	
Revenge	

■ Altered family relationships

The biggest loss when sexual abuse occurs in a family is the loss of innocence, of childhood and the loss of parents as good-enough father and mother.

When sexual abuse occurs between father and daughter, or father and son, the mother is usually in denial. This denial may be conscious, as in 'You're lying', or unconscious, as in 'I won't help you'. It may be important for the mother to keep the status quo. This leads her to collude with the abuser.

For reasons of her own, the mother may be unable to maintain a healthy sexual relationship with her partner and it therefore at some level suits her for the daughter or son to take on her sexual role. The scenario is complicated by the mother becoming a 'sibling', with the accompanying feelings of envy, jealousy and rivalry, often unconscious. The victim is effectively let down and abandoned by the one person she/he would turn to for help.

Denial and feelings of jealousy may also occur in the victim's sisters who consciously do not want to believe that their father is an abuser, but unconsciously may be angry at not being chosen.

■ Adult signs of childhood abuse

Adult victims of childhood abuse often show the symptoms of unresolved post-traumatic stress. They may suffer from serious problems such as:

- depression
- eating disorders
- body-image problems
- psychosomatic illnesses (in particular, gynaecological)
- self-harm
- suicide attempts.

They may behave in a seductive or provocative way. They may be angry or aggressive, or co-dependent, over-involved and over-accommodating. They may suffer from a fear of intimacy, difficulties in attachment, and difficulties with boundaries. They will find it difficult to allow themselves to be open, vulnerable and trusting.

While these signs may not indicate childhood sexual abuse, it is so widespread that it is important to keep it in mind.

Sexual dysfunctions are common in victims of childhood sexual abuse and include phobia, loss of desire, anorgasmia, vaginismus, dyspareunia in women and erectile difficulties in men (*see* Chapter 7).

Victims of sexual abuse use defence mechanisms such as:

- avoidance
- denial
- displacement
- disassociation
- repression
- splitting off.

This repeats the pattern of unconscious dynamics that the adults around them have acted out during the period of childhood abuse.

■ Disclosure

Whatever the therapist's personal opinion, it is essential that she does not jump to conclusions and suggest to the client that she/he may have been abused and has repressed the memory of the abuse, for the client may then confess to a false memory of abuse in order to please the therapist.

Disclosure is risky for the client, who may end the therapy to avoid the risk of experiencing overwhelmingly painful and shameful feelings. If the client is close to disclosure, the therapist must not be pushy or penetrative, thereby repeating the abuse. There needs to be a strong therapeutic alliance based on trust.

In couples therapy, disclosure of childhood sexual abuse can be a turning point in a relationship. If the couple's relationship itself is abusive, it may fall apart, but if it is strong enough, it can move forward.

Both partners may regress. The client may relive the original trauma and be flooded with sensory memories. The partner may feel hurt that the victim chose to reveal the abuse in therapy, and not personally to her/him.

The therapist needs to keep strong boundaries, be containing and safe and work sensitively and skilfully while remaining objective.

Sexual abuse is a murky and tricky area to work with because the client has experienced a different reality and major boundaries have been transgressed.

It arouses very primitive anxieties and leads to confused thinking. Speaking honestly and openly about it can be hard and often therapists feel de-skilled. It is more common than we may suppose.

■ Transference and countertransference

The transferential feelings and issues which may be projected onto the therapist by the victim of sexual abuse include:

- a desire to be special
- a chance to form a trusting relationship without the abuse being repeated
- a need to exert power, control
- love, hate
- a need to apportion blame, judgement
- seduction
- a tendency to intrude, probe, penetrate
- a need to test others or be tested oneself
- the desire for a good, healing parent.

Countertransferential feelings and issues which the therapist may project onto the client include.

- helplessness
- de-skilled

- overwhelmed
- anxiety
- disbelief
- revulsion
- anger
- fear
- revenge
- contamination
- resistance
- avoidance
- judgemental
- abused, abusive
- patronising
- paranoia
- pity
- rescuer
- protective
- parental
- curiosity
- fascination
- turned on
- unresolved personal issues.

Example: **'Daddy's girl'**

Larry and Denise had been married for over 20 years. She had married young to get away from home. Denise was ambivalent about staying in the relationship, although Larry was the only consistent and safe person in her life. She had had several affairs, which he had tolerated. She saw him as weak and needy, although he was caring and nurturing. Their relationship was co-dependent and collusive. (*See* Figure 6.1.)

She felt that her mother had abandoned her by going back to work when she was five. Her father sexually abused her until puberty. His attention made her feel special.

Her father, who was a swimming instructor, was arrested for abusing one of the children having swimming lessons when Denise was 20. She was very upset because she thought she was the only one. He had been unfaithful. Her feelings were split between disgust, anger, guilt and a loving desire to protect him.

When they came to counselling, her father was ill with cancer. Her relationship with him at this point was distant and polite. She had not forgiven him. Her promiscuity was as much an attack against him as it was a defence against intimacy with Larry.

Larry had been ill recently which reminded her of her father. She referred to him as lying in an unmade bed with a needy look, all messy and sweaty.

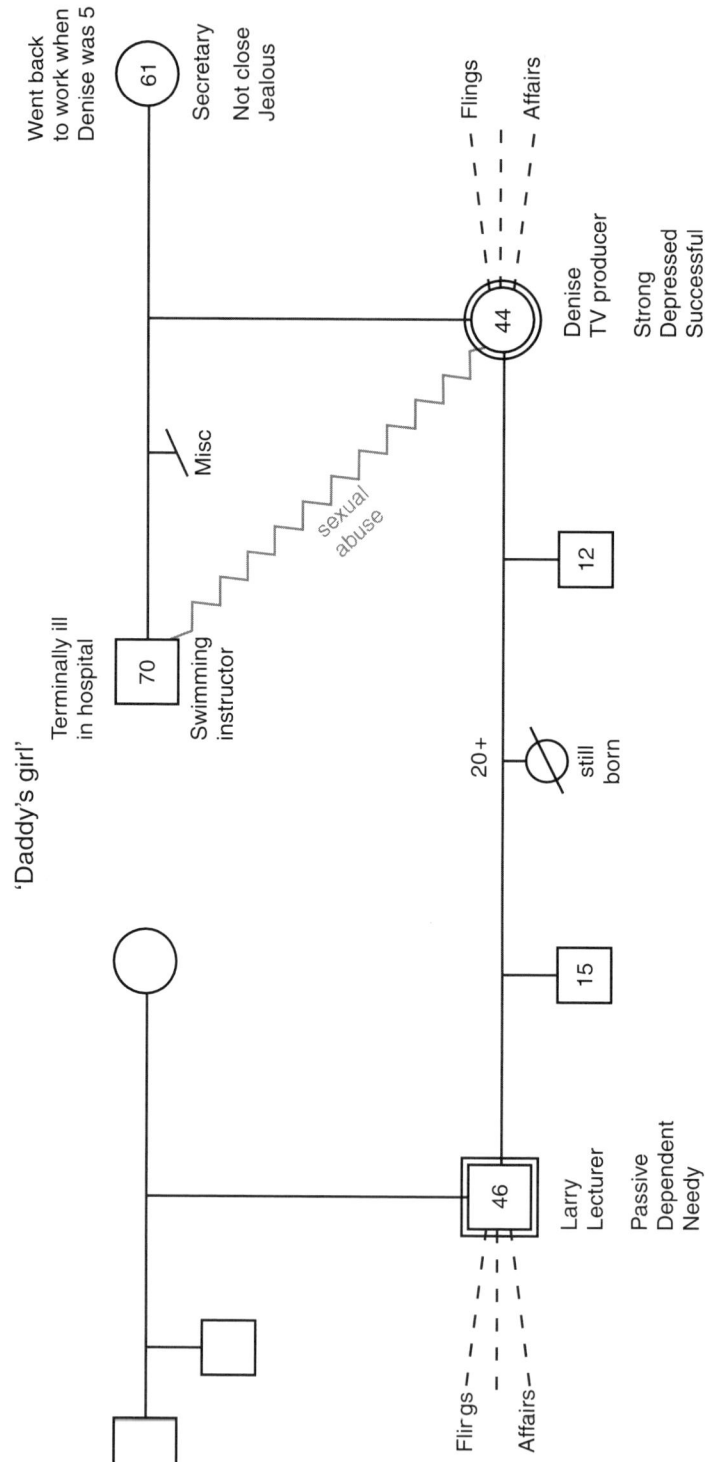

Figure 6.1 'Daddy's girl.'

> Denise wanted sex with Larry in settings other than the bedroom that were novel and exciting, so that it felt like an affair. Her father came to her bedroom during her childhood. In her inner world her father was her primary partner, the love of her life.
>
> Denise went to visit her father after a long gap. He died soon after. She felt angry and guilty but relieved. Her murderous feelings were projected onto Larry for a while, but she also felt a strong sexual energy towards him. She stopped flirting with other men and started owning the losses that she had undergone by being in an incestuous relationship. Slowly she moved towards a deeper and more intimate commitment to the marriage and was able to acknowledge Larry's love for her.
>
> Denise dominated the therapy, which is reflected in this account. In the countertransference I felt de-skilled, challenged, and not quite good enough. I did not always feel in control. It was difficult knowing what was real and what was fantasy.
>
> Although Denise and Larry had reached some kind of accommodation in their relationship, it was clear that Denise's father had been the love of her life and always would be.

There is a general reluctance to confront the problems of sexual abuse because they touch primitive and fearful parts of our unconscious. Yet therapists need to be very aware of sexual abuse as it is very common in the clients who present for therapy.

■ Paraphilias

Paraphilias are recurrent sexually arousing fantasies, sexual urges or behaviours generally involving objects, suffering or humiliation of oneself or partner, or children and non-consenting persons.

Paraphilias can arouse a degree of curiosity in the therapist, a form of projected fascination in the client's unusual behaviour. Occurrence of paraphilias in couples work is infrequent. It is almost always a male phenomenon. The most common ones in the context of a relationship are:

* masochism
* sadism
* transvestism
* fetishism.

And more rarely:

* paedophilia
* voyeurism
* exhibitionism
* frotteurism.

The focus of the work with couples is usually about the other partner's ability and willingness to tolerate the paraphilia. The paraphilic may make some temporary behavioural changes but is rarely motivated to give up the acting out of his fantasy altogether.

■ Definitions

- *Masochism*: Desire to be humiliated, beaten, bound or otherwise made to suffer.
- *Sadism*: When psychological or physical suffering of a victim is sexually exciting.
- *Transvestism*: Desire in heterosexual or homosexual men to wear women's clothing.
- *Fetishism*: The use of objects for arousing desire.
- *Paedophilia*: Desire for sexual activity with a pre-pubescent child.
- *Voyeurism*: Observing an unsuspecting person who is undressing, naked or involved in sexual activity.
- *Exhibitionism*: Exposing one's genitals to an unsuspecting stranger.
- *Frotteurism*: Touching or rubbing against a non-consenting person.

Example: **'Silk knickers'**

Paraphilics are notoriously resistant to change and loath to give up their compulsive behaviour. In couples work the focus is on whether the partner can accept and tolerate the fetishistic behaviour without it feeling like a collusive co-dependence or a defeat.

Terry and Julie came for therapy because Terry was a transvestite and Julie was fed up with it. She did not mind dressing up in soft creamy lingerie and stockings for him but she hated seeing him in women's clothing. (*See* Figure 6.2.)

Terry was the youngest of four, the only boy, and his mother's favourite. His father had abandoned the family soon after his birth. His mother kept him in her bed until he went to primary school. She walked about the house in her underwear. She wore silk nighties and soft underwear, always in pastel colours. She would ask Terry to help her dress. At night in bed he would snuggle up to her and revel in her sensual warmth and the texture of her nightie. In adolescence, Terry took a pair of her knickers out of her chest of drawers and used them for masturbation. Eventually he started wearing them when he masturbated.

Terry knew Julie from school. They started dating when they were 16 and were soon having sex together. Julie was really surprised when Terry bought her underwear and did not mind wearing it for sex. Even when he started wearing it 'for fun' she went along with him. They married when they were 19.

Julie and Terry worked in a local hairdresser's. Terry inherited some money from his grandfather and bought into the business. Eventually he became a partner and Julie was the salon manager.

Terry's office opened up onto the salon. He loved working there, next to the hum of the dryers, the swish of silky wraps, the smell of shampoo, the sound of women's voices. He loved women. Dressing as a woman both thrilled and soothed him. Under the skirt inside the silk knickers was his secret weapon, his erect penis. He wanted to cross-dress at work, but he knew Julie would not allow it.

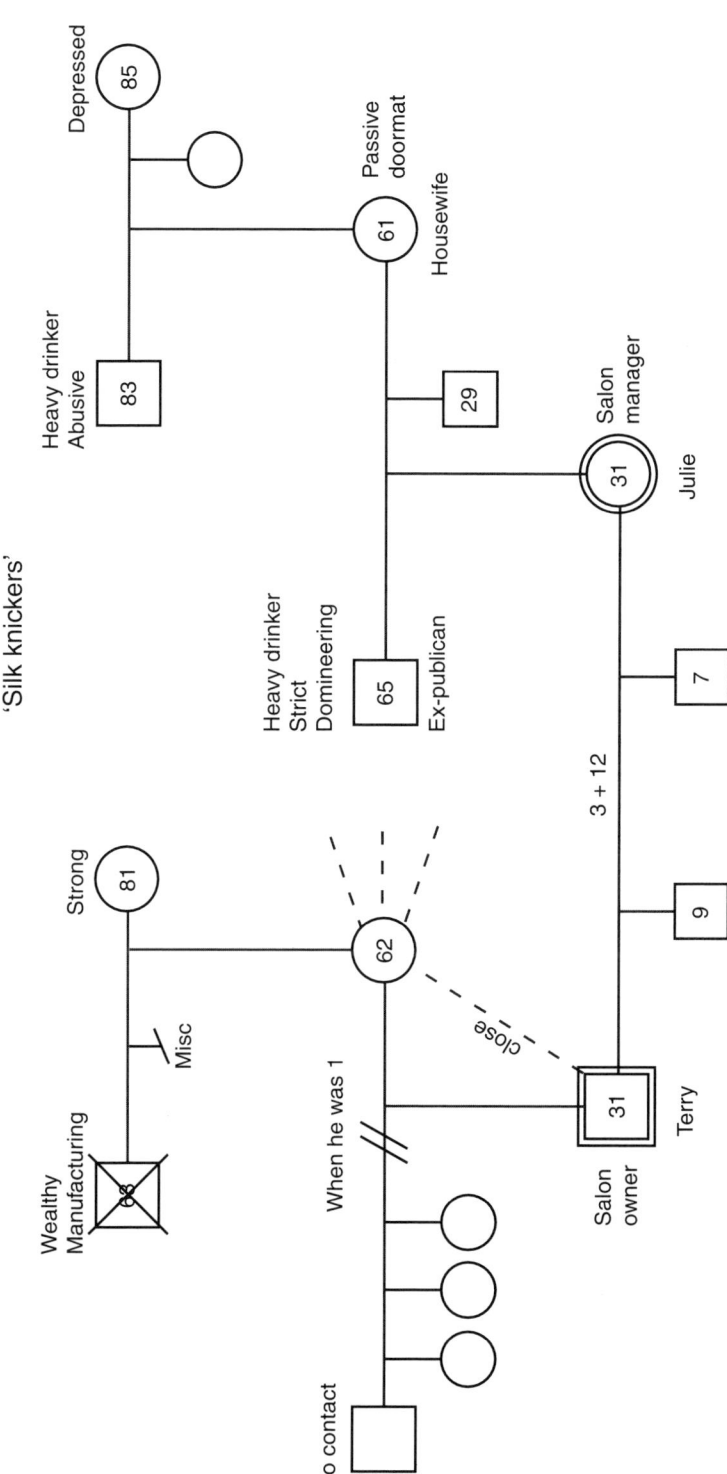

Figure 6.2 'Silk knickers.'

Julie was ashamed. She had protected the children from Terry's habit, but she feared he was getting bolder. She did not want him to go out in public dressed as a woman. She knew Terry was fantasising about it.

Julie had come from a family of passive, compliant women who did what they were told. She was determined not to be a doormat like her mother. She was attracted to Terry because of his feminine side. He would not tell her what to do. But he exercised his power over her in another way. Julie was realistic. The business was going well, money problems had eased. Terry was a caring father. Sex was literally a bit of a performance, but they loved each other.

They came to a compromise. Terry promised never to go public or cross-dress in front of the children. Julie accepted with difficulty that he would not give up his habit. My concern was that the agreement would not hold. Terry would eventually want the thrill of being out in the world dressed up as a woman. Would Julie put up with it or would she leave? My guess was that she would put up with it because her experience was that that was what women do.

■ Sexual addiction

If a client is using compulsive sex as an escape from unbearable feelings and feels anxious without frequent sex, then one can start to think of her/his behaviour in terms of addiction. This applies to masturbatory and paraphilic activity as well.

Some of the vocabulary associated with eating disorders can also apply to sexual behaviour.

■ Sexual bulimia

This is a repetitive pattern of sexual binge and guilt with an associated search for comfort and relief.

Men: Men who are addicted to sex very often have had cold, unloving mothers who have rejected or abandoned them. The unconscious fantasy is of somehow finding through repeated sexual connection the missing emotional connection to the unavailable or absent mother. The power of the penis may also be a way of persecuting and punishing the bad mother and women in general.

Example: Hugh Hefner, the founder of *Playboy* magazine and a hugely successful sex industry, is never without two or three busty young blondes by his side and in his bed. He once said in an interview that he did not have a single memory of being hugged or touched by his mother.

Women: Women with a compulsive need for sex are generally using their bodies as a way of getting their emotional needs met. They are looking for:

• attention
• attachment
• affection
• approval
• reassurance

- regard
- intimacy.

Their behaviour is often manipulative and neurotic. It usually results in rejection by their sexual partners, who are unwilling or unable to give them what they really need. This increases their sense of worthlessness, which feeds their destructive behaviour and sexual acting out.

These women are frequently the daughters of distant or unavailable fathers and have never been validated by a safe man as attractive young women. They are looking for comfort and affirmation through sex.

Example: Marilyn Monroe never knew her father. Her schizophrenic mother was hospitalised during her childhood and she was fostered, sexually abused and put in an orphanage. She married her first husband at 16. She called Arthur Miller, her third husband, 'Daddy'. She wanted to be taken seriously as an actress but is remembered as a sexual icon (*see* Figure 6.3).

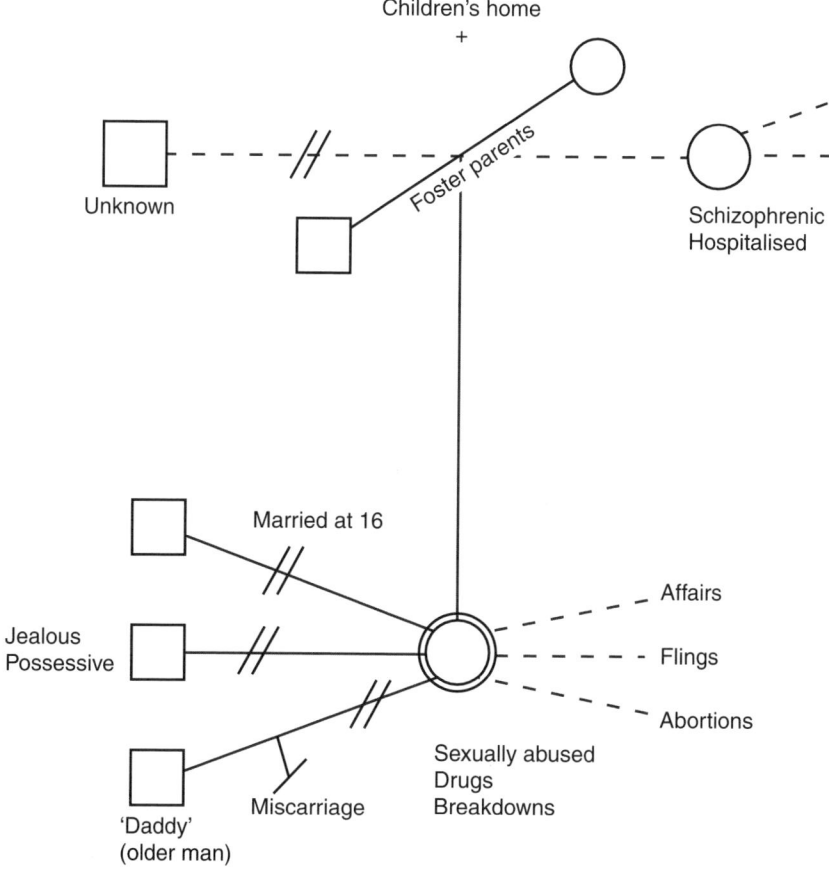

Figure 6.3 Genogram: Marilyn Monroe.

The feelings shared by male and female sex addicts include:

- worthlessness
- low self-esteem
- guilt
- shame
- anxiety
- emotional deprivation
- destructiveness to self and partners
- desire to punish
- search for reparation.

■ Sexual anorexia

The causes of sexual anorexia are many. It is not merely loss of desire, low libido or lack of appetite. Sex may be avoided because of strong childhood messages of guilt or shame, or religious strictures that make sex sinful or dirty.

The power of sexuality may have been experienced in the family as dangerous and may therefore be repressed and inhibited.

Bad experiences such as abuse, assault, rape, unwanted pregnancy, termination or sexually transmitted disease can lead to sexual anorexia.

The incest taboo and a failure to work through Oedipal issues will affect the sexual appetite. The inability to detach from the opposite-sex parent at an unconscious level, when sex is present but forbidden, can lead to a deeply entrenched fear of sex, even in legitimate adult relationships.

Just as an anorexic finds a sense of power and control in refusing food, so does the partner who withholds sex. Sex is used as a currency, or a reward, and becomes a bargaining tool in a continuing power struggle and battle for control.

Example: **'Addicted to sex'**

Cliff was a sex addict. He lived with his partner but he was also in two ongoing relationships and he had flings on the side. (*See* Figure 6.4.)

Cliff was the manager of a shoe shop, so he met new women every day. Juggling his sexual relationships was time-consuming and caused him a lot of anxiety, but the rush of excitement made it worthwhile. He came to therapy because he had fallen in love and he did not know how to give up his addiction to sex.

He had been with his partner, Marilyn, for some years, but ironically they had stopped having sex. She was the stability in his life. She provided a home, a safe place for him, but she was not a warm, giving person.

His other relationship was with a married woman, Shirley, whom he had known all his life. They had a warm physical relationship. Cliff confided in her and she never judged him. They got together every couple of weeks or so.

Then there was Cheryl. Cheryl was in love with Cliff and would do anything to please him. This included being at his beck and call and acting out his sexual fantasies. Cheryl had dressed up, been tied up, had sex in public places, been used and abused, but she still loved him.

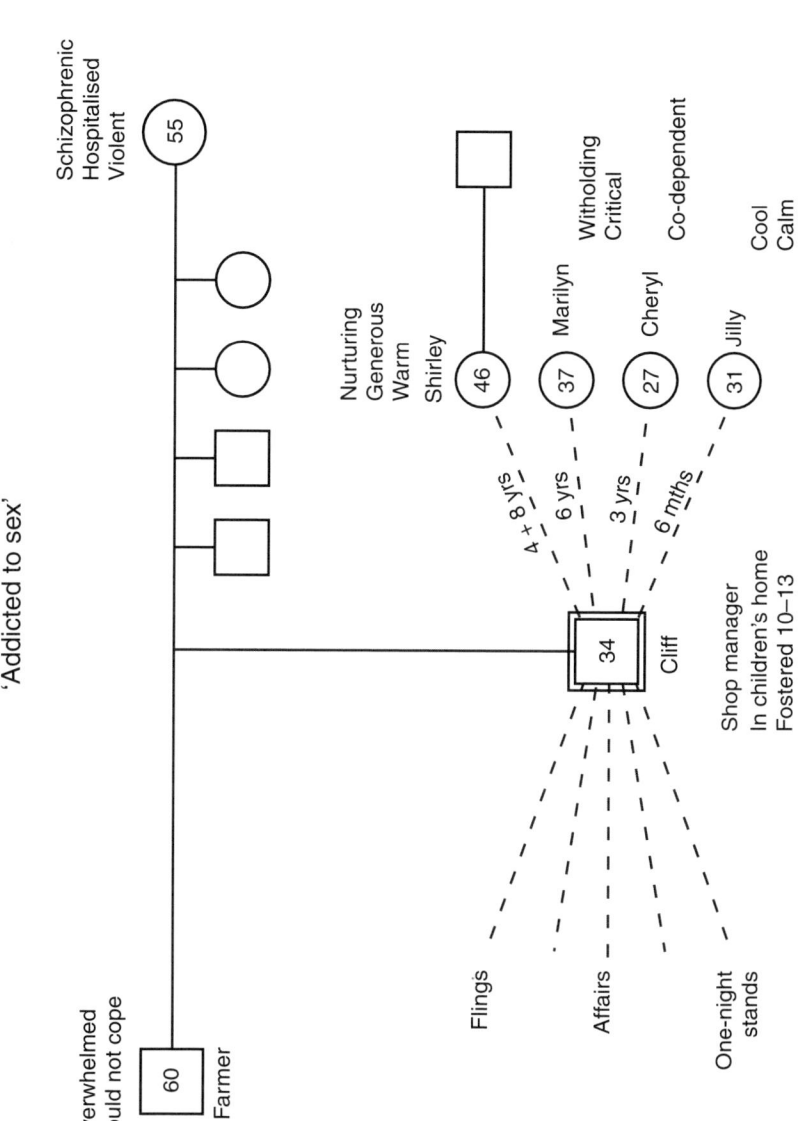

Figure 6.4 'Addicted to sex.'

Like all addicts, Cliff was trying to fill the emptiness within and keep depression at bay. If he did not have sexual intercourse at least once a day the panic would rise in him.

And now he had met Jilly, who worked in a doctor's practice. Jilly had not succumbed to his charms, which made him want her all the more. Her unavailability made him feel desolate and rejected.

Cliff was the oldest of five children. His mother was in and out of psychiatric hospitals throughout his childhood. His father, who was a farmer, could not cope and had put the children in care. Cliff had lived in a home between the ages of five and seven. He had been fostered for three years, aged ten to 13, and had left home at 16. He had been an emotional orphan from the age of five and he missed his mother and the mothering he had never had. Sex was a defence against anxiety and depression, a search for a connection with the abandoning, unavailable mother.

In the classic 'mother/Madonna/whore' split (*see* p. 24), Marilyn and Shirley were maternal figures, one withholding, one giving. Cheryl and his flings were the sexual objects and Jilly was the idealised, pure, unobtainable one.

I had to be able to tolerate all these projections in the transference. Cliff tried to seduce me for months. It started with invitations for a drink or a meal. He sent me e-mails. He asked me to visit him at home when Marilyn was away. He paid me compliments about my looks, my appearance, my clothes. Finally he came out with it straight: would I go to bed with him? 'No' was my answer. He told me how relieved he was and the real work started after that.

It took a long time for Cliff to trust me. He tested me endlessly. I had to keep very firm boundaries, not be judgemental or critical, and show him enough concern, respect and positive regard for him to begin to feel he could be a worthwhile human being. Exploring Cliff's childhood was a very painful experience for him. Slowly he began to understand what had happened to him and why he acted out sexually.

■ The sexual assessment and genogram

Making a sexual assessment in the context of couples therapy is factual, focused and detailed. The assessment will provide a full sexual history of each partner and their sexual difficulties within the context of their families. Because it is a directive process, one or other partner, or both, may show anxiety, reluctance and avoidance, and will need reassurance.

The therapist needs to work intuitively. She cannot expect to get answers to all the questions in one session. The following list is a framework. While discussing the issues listed with each partner, the therapist will also learn from the partners' interaction, communication style and body language as each topic is explored.

■ Presenting problem
- Description.
- Duration.

- Why do the partners think they have a problem?
- What makes it better?
- Treatments so far?
- Is it present in different situations?
- What is the couple's expectation of therapy?

■ History of the relationship

- Duration.
- Married or living together.
- Children, miscarriages, terminations.
- Previous marriages and important relationships.
- Divorces.
- Quality of relationship.
- Communication of feelings.
- How anger and conflict are dealt with.

■ Medical history

- Medication (prescribed or other), contraception.
- Cigarettes, alcohol and drug consumption.
- Illness, operations, accidents.

■ Childhood experience and key events

- Quality of parents' relationship.
- Divorces in family.
- Family atmosphere.
- Mental illnesses, addictions.
- Siblings.
- How anger was expressed.
- Schooling – parental attitudes to achievement.
- Was sex openly discussed?
- An easy-going or strict atmosphere.
- Parental attitudes to sex.
- Affection between parents and siblings.
- Religious or cultural upbringing.

■ Sexual development

- Sex education and knowledge.
- Pleasant and unpleasant sexual experiences.
- Menstruation, wet dreams.
- Masturbation, orgasm, ejaculation.
- Dating.

- Homosexual experiences.
- First sexual encounter.
- First sexual intercourse.
- Sexual enjoyment.
- Guilt about sex.

■ Current sexual activity

- Sexual practices and preferences.
- Frequency of sexual contact and intercourse.
- Positions.
- Inhibitions and embarrassment.
- Foreplay and sexual caressing.
- Oral sex.
- Anal sex.
- Fantasies.
- Turn-ons and offs.
- Use of sex aids.
- Masturbation.
- Satisfaction, orgasm.

■ Lifestyle, values and beliefs

- Religious and cultural beliefs and attitudes.
- Experience of violence.
- Experience of sexual abuse.
- Affairs.
- Social life and work.
- Body image and self-confidence.
- Bereavements.

■ Questions to ask

- What happens when you have sex?
- When was the last time you made love?
- Was that typical of your recent sexual experiences together?
- How often do you make love?
- Where did you make love?
- Is that usually where you have sex?
- What time of day was it?
- Were you dressed or undressed; what were you wearing?
- Was it light or dark?
- Who initiated sex?
- Who usually initiates?
- How do you let each other know when you are interested in sex?

- How do you react when your partner approaches you?
- Do you know what each other likes sexually?
- Do you know what you like?
- How absorbed do you become in making love?

■ Exploring the sexual genogram

The process of building a genogram should start with requests for information and clarification of family experiences.

Working with the clients' apprehensions and concerns in a sexual context requires respect and tact. There needs to be a reflective review of the process, a look at how the couple can apply what they have learned about each other to their sexual relationship and its difficulties. The genogram forms the basis for these discussions.

The following questions are asked of each partner in turn and discussed in the sessions. This is best done informally.

- What are/were the overt/covert messages in your family regarding sexuality/intimacy?
- … And regarding masculinity/femininity?
- Who said what/did what? Who was conspicuously silent/absent in the area of sexuality/intimacy?
- Who was the most open sexually or intimately and in what ways?
- How were sexuality and intimacy encouraged? Discouraged? Controlled? Within a generation? Between generations?
- What questions regarding sexuality/intimacy in your family tree have you been reluctant to ask? Who might have the answers? How could you discover the answers?
- What were the 'secrets' in your family regarding sexuality/intimacy, e.g. incest, unwanted pregnancies, extra-marital affairs?
- What do other family members have to say regarding the above questions? How did these issues, events, and experiences affect her/him? Within a generation? Between generations? With whom have you talked about this? With whom would you like to talk about it?
- How does your partner perceive your family tree regarding these issues? How do you perceive hers/his?
- How would you change this genogram (including who and what) to meet your wishes of what could have occurred regarding messages and experiences of sexuality and intimacy?

Example: **Duncan and Susie**

Duncan and Susie came for therapy because she suffered from dyspareunia (painful intercourse). They were trying for a baby, but hardly having any sex.

By going through the assessment process and building a sexual genogram, the following emerged. (*See* Figure 6.5.)

Susie had always experienced pain on intercourse. She felt guilty and disappointed about the lack of sex. She also suffered from chronic thrush, which she self-medicated because she was too embarrassed to talk to the doctor.

Her previous relationships had never lasted more than a year because of the sexual difficulties. Sex was less painful when she had had a few drinks, but she never really enjoyed it and had never had an orgasm. She did not masturbate. She had had a miscarriage in the previous year and was still very sad about it.

Feelings were not shown in her family and sex was never talked about. She was close to her mother and described her father as distant. Her mother had given her very negative messages about childbirth and had told her that 'doing it' was something you had to put up with if you wanted to have a baby.

Duncan also felt guilty and disappointed. In order not to hurt Susie he ejaculated as quickly as possible. He admitted that he had always done that and his previous relationship had ended because the sex was unsatisfactory and had stopped. They generally used condoms, which made Susie's thrush worse, but this was a problem they had not discussed. Duncan too was sad about the lost baby but had not talked about it.

Duncan's brother was successful, as was his father. They were competitive and argumentative as a family, with high expectations of achievement. Duncan had self-esteem issues and felt he had not done well enough.

Susie and Duncan presented with a specific sexual dysfunction (hers). Yet the assessment provided a very full picture of what might be problematic in the relationship for both of them.

I felt we could work both psychosexually and psychodynamically. I started with a mutually agreed ban on sexual intercourse to take away any pressure, anxiety or expectation. I suggested that they both do self-focus exercises and talk about it in the sessions. We looked at the emotional climate in both their families and what gender and sexual messages they had each received.

They mourned their lost baby together and shared their hopes about having another one. We explored their shared loss of self-esteem and feelings of guilt and disappointment.

Doing a sexual genogram proved to be a rich way into some really useful work.

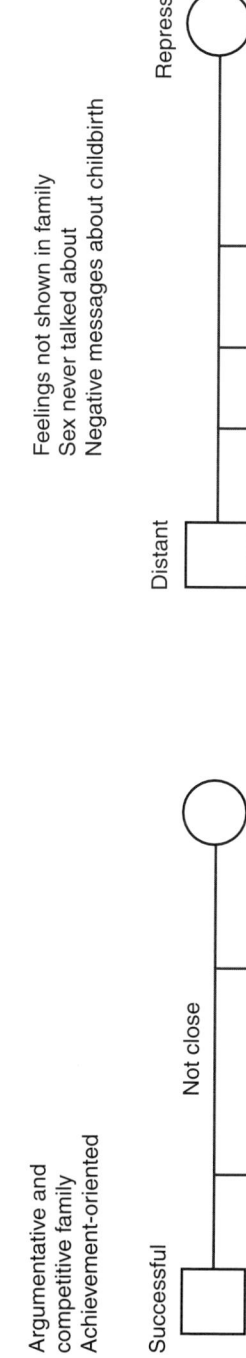

Figure 6.5 Genogram: Duncan and Susie.

CHAPTER 7

No sex

Bad sex leads to no sex. Sexual activity between couples ceases when sexual problems become unmanageable. The causes of 'no sex' are many but this remains an area that many therapists are understandably nervous about. Add that to the clients' embarrassment and the sexual problems may not be addressed in a way that is helpful to the couple.

■ The causes of 'no sex'

The causes of 'no sex' are a range of sexual dysfunctions.

- Male   – erectile disorder
        – premature ejaculation
        – retarded ejaculation
        – loss of desire.
- Female – inorgasmia
        – dyspareunia
        – vaginismus
        – loss of desire.

Sexual dysfunctions can have physical or psychological origins, or a combination of both. The physical causes of sexual dysfunctions include:

- illness
- trauma
- injury
- surgery
- pain
- disability
- addiction
- exhaustion
- ME
- depression
- medication
- infertility
- pregnancy
- childbirth.

The psychological causes can be interpersonal (to do with the relationship) or intra-personal (to do with the individual), and may be further categorised as predisposing, precipitating or perpetuating (*see* Figure 7.1).

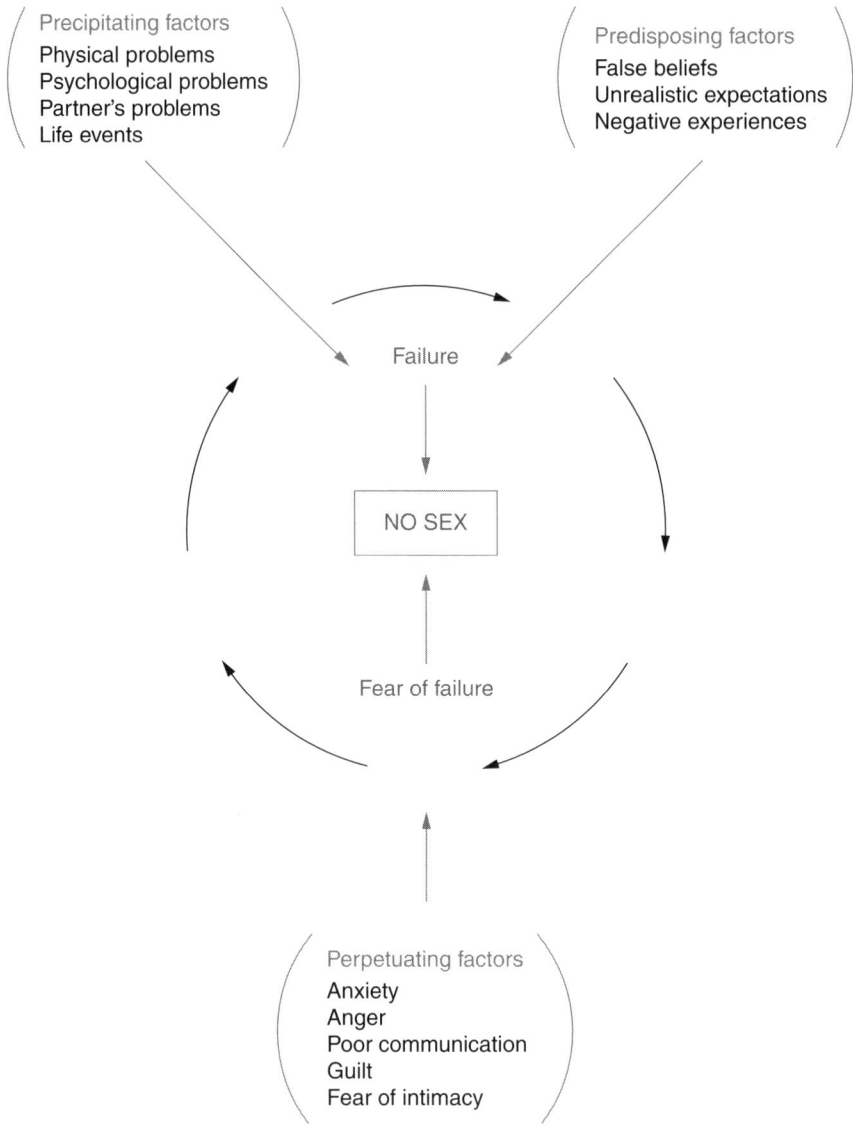

Figure 7.1   Psychological causes of no sex.

■ Predisposing factors

These are conscious and unconscious messages acquired in childhood and are caused by:

- ignorance
- repressive upbringing
- taboos
- incest
- false expectations

- false beliefs
- abuse
- rape
- gender issues
- stereotyping.

■ Precipitating factors

These arise from life events and crises such as:

- illness
- childbirth
- trauma
- unemployment
- redundancy
- affairs
- unreasonable expectations
- partner's sexual dysfunctions
- failure
- depression.

■ Perpetuating factors

These result from the sexual dysfunction itself or the relationship in which the sexual dysfunction has occurred, and include:

- anxiety leading to performance anxiety, anticipatory failure and avoidance
- anger, criticism, rows
- poor communication
- fear of intimacy
- fear of commitment
- guilt and shame.

When one partner in the couple presents with a sexual dysfunction, the therapist needs to look to the other partner to see what the collusive fit may be. For example, the partner of a man with erectile problems or premature ejaculation may often be suffering from dyspareunia (pain on intercourse). There is a shared avoidance of intercourse, which protects her as well as him from sexual activity.

Ideally, psychosexual therapy is done with the couple. However, a client may present with a sexual problem on her/his own for the following reasons:

- The partner has gone.
- The client does not want the partner to attend.
- The partner refuses to come.
- The client is presenting with a primary problem.
- The client is not in a relationship.

Psychosexual work with a single client would include a sexual assessment and formulation, self-focus exercises, exploration of fantasies, and reframing of negative messages (*see* Chapter 5). The therapist needs to keep firm boundaries and be very aware of the transference and countertransference when working with a single client.

■ Male sexual dysfunctions

■ Erectile disorder

Definition: Persistent or recurrent inability to attain or maintain an adequate erection until completion of the sexual activity.

Areas to be explored
1 Check medical history for:
- diabetes
- cardiovascular problems
- multiple sclerosis
- accidents, trauma or injury
- medication
- testosterone levels
- long-term use of alcohol and nicotine.
2 Check early family experiences and messages about sex.
3 Check feelings about personal sexuality and gender identity.
4 Check adolescent fantasies and first experience of sex.
5 Check for fear of penetration. Is it seen as a violent or abusive act? Is there a fear of the engulfing vagina?
6 Check for incest taboo. Was the mother possessive, intrusive and overwhelming?
7 Check for recent losses such as bereavement, redundancy, divorce, also loss of professional or personal role and status, disappointment, failure.
8 Check for mid-life crisis, expectations of ageing, body image.
9 Check for current relationship and family problems.

If the man achieves a spontaneous morning erection on waking or on masturbation, the causes of his erectile problems are more likely to be psychological than physical.

When working with couples where the man has sexual dysfunction it is important to look at the problem in the context of the relationship and whether the partner has sexual problems also.

If the man has not fully separated from his mother during his Oedipal phase, he may unconsciously split off his fears of incest and project them onto his penis. Women are identified with the mother and are not seen as sexual partners. The incest taboo is stronger than desire. Erectile failure protects him from actual intercourse.

If there has been no intercourse in the relationship for a period of time, the couple may need to talk about the implications of change.

Working behaviourally, the first aim would be to eliminate performance anxiety and the partner's expectations so that there are no demands or any pressure to achieve an erection. The sensate focus exercises (described later) are particularly effective for erectile disorder in the context of couples therapy. It might be appropriate to give the man self-focus exercises at the same time.

If he is considering practical help, he needs to consult his GP, especially if he is considering a drug such as Viagra. This drug works by controlling one enzyme that acts on a second enzyme, which expands the veins in the penis. This is why Viagra does not work unless there is desire and a signal from the brain to release the first enzyme. Second generation drugs such as Levitra are now available.

Erections can also be achieved with the use of a vacuum pump or papaverine injections into the penis.

If he has had erectile dysfunction for a long time and is suddenly able to perform again, the partner's feelings need to be explored. She may not be so willing to restart sexual intercourse.

Example: 'Let's not do it'

Phil and Anita had been together for five years. Two years into the relationship Anita lost her job and caught a very nasty flu virus, which turned into ME. This lasted for 18 months, during which time Phil looked after her with much devotion. Their sexual relationship was fine until Anita fell ill. When she started to feel better and they wanted to resume their sexual activity Phil developed erection difficulties at the moment of penetration. There was a lot of shared foreplay and mutual masturbation, but Anita wanted full penetrative sex. Phil felt a failure and Anita felt confused. (*See* Figure 7.2.)

Doing a sexual assessment was very informative. Phil's mother had breast cancer and was exhausted by her chemotherapy treatment.

When Phil was 18 his sister had had a near-fatal car accident and had spent three months in hospital. Phil had been a good carer. His experience of the women he loved was that they were vulnerable and fragile. And now Anita had joined them.

Anita's parents had divorced when she was ten. Her father had remarried and had two new daughters. Anita felt neglected. He had never made her feel special. She was very close to her mother, who was rather controlling. Phil had helped to give her a lot of confidence, but with her illness she had lost some of her self-esteem. She was concerned that Phil did not really desire her, which would explain why he could not maintain his erection. It turned out that when they had resumed their sexual relationship she had felt pain on intercourse. Anita was embarrassed to talk about this because she felt a failure. Neither of them saw the other as fully functioning sexual beings and they had both got stuck with this perception. She was an invalid; he was her nurse. He did not want to cause her pain on penetration. She did not want him to feel bad about his loss of erection. There was an unconscious collusive avoidance of intercourse. Working psychodynamically and behaviourally with this couple was very helpful. They enjoyed the sensate focus exercises, which enabled them to be close and intimate without any pressure, and they gained a lot of insight into their relationship. Eventually Phil stopped worrying about his erection and Anita relaxed. After a while they were able to have penetrative sex without an absolute goal.

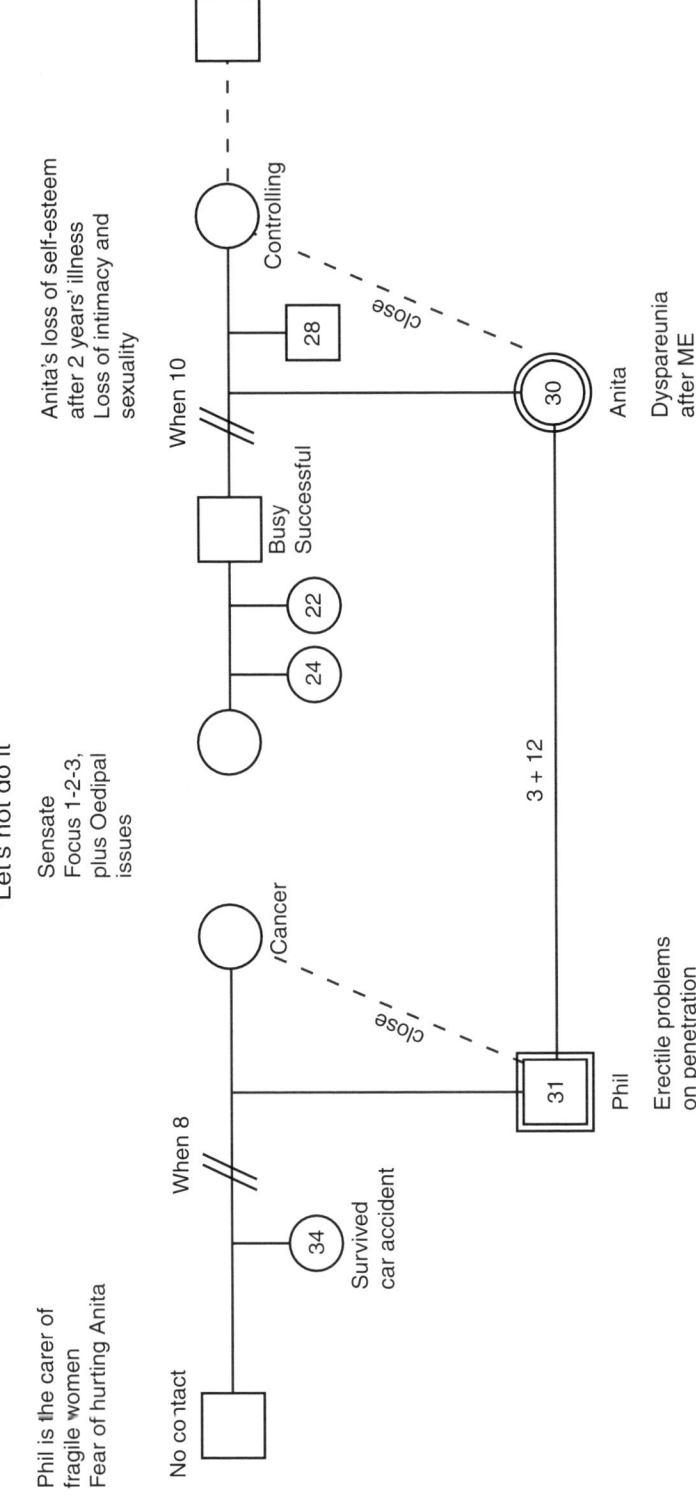

Figure 7.2 'Let's not do it.'

■ Premature ejaculation

Definition: Persistent or recurrent ejaculation with minimal sexual stimulation before or shortly after penetration and before it is wished for.

Areas to be explored
1 Does he have any control over ejaculation during masturbation, foreplay or penetration?
2 What are his masturbatory techniques?
3 Is there any guilt about sex or issues with his personal sexuality?
4 Is there a history of bedwetting?
5 What were his adolescent relationships like?
6 Are there any reasons for anxiety and an inability to relax?
7 Are there power struggles and battles for control in the relationship?
8 Does it suit the partner not to have full intercourse?

Premature ejaculation is about not recognising the cut-off point of ejaculatory inevitability. The man goes from foreplay to ejaculation with virtually no plateau phase.

The behavioural intervention called the squeeze technique is very effective. The man presses his thumb down hard on top of the penile ridge when he feels he is close to ejaculating. This will keep him in the plateau phase. The exercise is repeated three times in succession. It can then be done by the partner on subsequent occasions. When he is confident about recognising the point of inevitability he may try the stop/start technique with vaginal containment, as described on p. 157.

■ Retarded ejaculation

Definition: Persistent or recurrent delay in or absence of ejaculation during sexual activity.

Areas to be explored
1 Use of medications, in particular anti-depressants.
2 Spinal injuries.
3 Is there a history of bedwetting?
4 Is there a fear of letting go, losing control?
5 Has there been any sexual abuse?
6 Be sensitive to his religious background.
7 Are his masturbatory practices very vigorous?
8 Consider his relationship with his mother (*see* p. 144).

Retarded ejaculation is not very common, but is quite difficult to treat. If the man does not ejaculate when masturbating, relaxation and self-focus exercises are helpful.

Masturbation by the partner and use of fantasy would be the next step. When that is successful, he can introduce the penis into the vagina just before ejaculating. This may need to be repeated several times on different occasions to allay his fears of vaginal engulfment (*see* p. 144).

It is worth exploring the client's attitude to women. Does he have an underlying anger and hostility? Withholding may be a way of punishing his partner, onto whom he has projected his unconscious negative feelings about women.

■ Female sexual dysfunctions

■ Inorgasmia

Definition: Absence of orgasm following sexual activity.

Areas to be explored
1 Does she experience desire and arousal?
2 Can she reach orgasm when she masturbates?
3 Can she reach orgasm when her partner stimulates her manually or orally?
4 Does she have an expectation of being orgasmic during intercourse?
5 What were the family messages about sex, in particular from her mother?
6 Be sensitive to her religious background.
7 Check for traumas in her past.
8 Is there a fear of letting go, losing control?

With a combination of relaxation and self-focus exercises, she can then progress to masturbation with the use of fantasy.

Some women find themselves able to let go if they role-play having an orgasm through breathing and movement.

Finally, the use of a vibrator is usually very successful because of the level of clitoral stimulation it provides.

Communication with her partner is obviously very important so that their expectations of sex are shared and they both learn what is helpful.

Because the female orgasm starts in the clitoris, the majority of women are not orgasmic during sexual intercourse.

■ Dyspareunia

Definition: Recurrent or persistent genital pain associated with sexual intercourse.

Areas to be explored
1 Physical causes need to be eliminated. These include:
  • vaginal infections
  • thrush
  • chlamydia
  • herpes
  • endometriosis
  • pelvic inflammatory disease
  • cystitis
  • post-natal or post-operative scarring
  • ovarian cysts.
2 Is she lubricating sufficiently?

3 Is she sensitive or allergic to soaps?
4 Can she use a tampon?
5 Has she been sexually abused?
6 Is she afraid of penetration?
7 Is she afraid of becoming pregnant?
8 Does she have fears about the size of her vagina and his penis?
9 Does she feel guilty about having sex?
10 Has she separated sufficiently from her mother?

■ Vaginismus

Definition: Recurrent or persistent involuntary spasm of the muscles of the outer third of the vagina, preventing intercourse.

Areas to be explored
1 Ask yourself if she may have been sexually abused.
2 How was her first period dealt with?
3 Can she use a tampon?
4 Is she concerned that her vagina may be too small?
5 Is she afraid of becoming pregnant?
6 Does she experience desire and arousal?
7 Does she come from an over-protected background?
8 Be sensitive to her religious background.
9 Did she feel rejected by her father at puberty?
10 What was her mother's view of sex?
11 Has she had negative experiences of sex?

Both dyspareunia and vaginismus respond to relaxation and self-focus exercises followed by sensate focus (*see* p. 155).

Eventually she can start to introduce her finger into the vagina, then two fingers. When she feels confident, she can ask her partner to introduce his finger, then two fingers.

The psychodynamic theory about dyspareunia and vaginismus is that there has been over-identification with the mother and no rivalry for the father during the Oedipal phase. This can lead to an inability to separate from the mother in later life. If the father has rejected her as a sexual being, there will be a conflict between desire and rejection, a struggle for autonomy, a need for sexual empowerment. She has to feel control over her body and her genitals. But there is a fear of being taken over and invaded (by the penis). The physical boundary of the vagina also represents a psychological boundary; it is her inner space. Unconscious split-off feelings are somatised and expressed physically in the vagina as tension, pain and muscular spasm (*see* Figure 7.3).

These symptoms are part of a defence against the anxiety of giving up the mother/baby bond for an adult sexual bond, of transforming an infantile attachment into a mature attachment and integrating the vagina with the body as a whole.

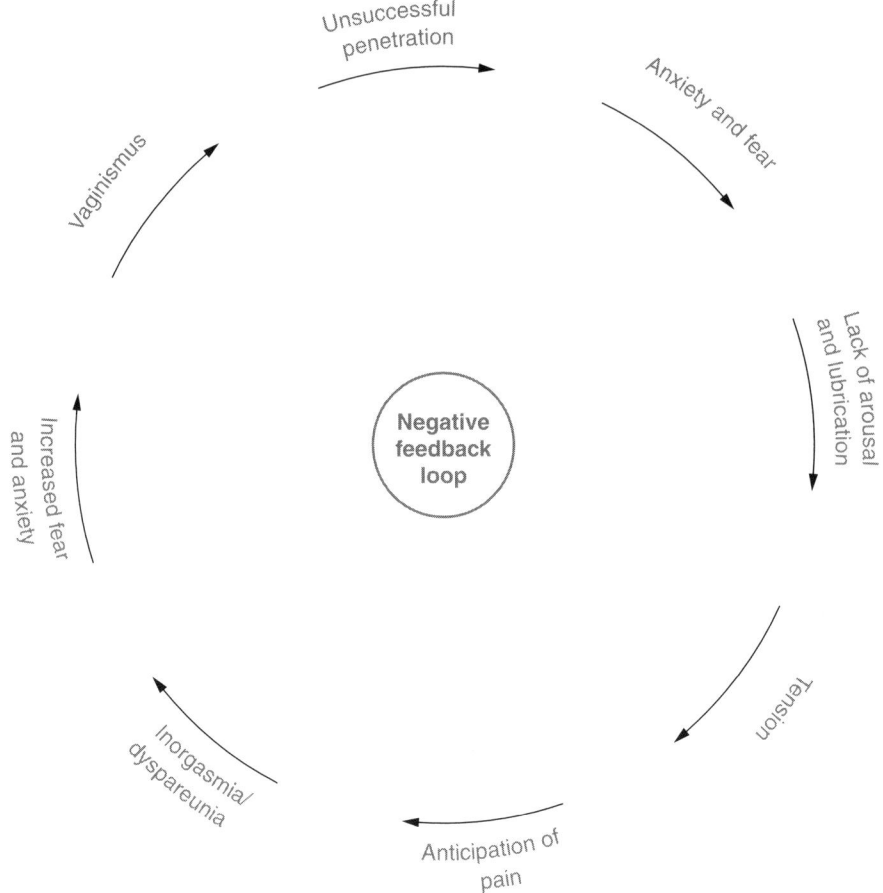

Figure 7.3   Negative feedback loop of female sexual dysfunctions.

Example: 'Daddy, don't go'

Amanda suffered from vaginismus and had had two relationships that had
ended because of her sexual difficulty. The first man had called her a freak,
and the second one had left her feeling a failure and convinced that she was
unattractive. She had not wanted sex with either of them, but did not know
how to say 'No' – her body had said it for her. (*See* Figure 7.4.)

Amanda's mother had had two miscarriages before Amanda was born and
had always told Amanda that another pregnancy would have killed her. Her
parents had not had sex since her birth. Amanda's understanding was that
sex was dangerous.

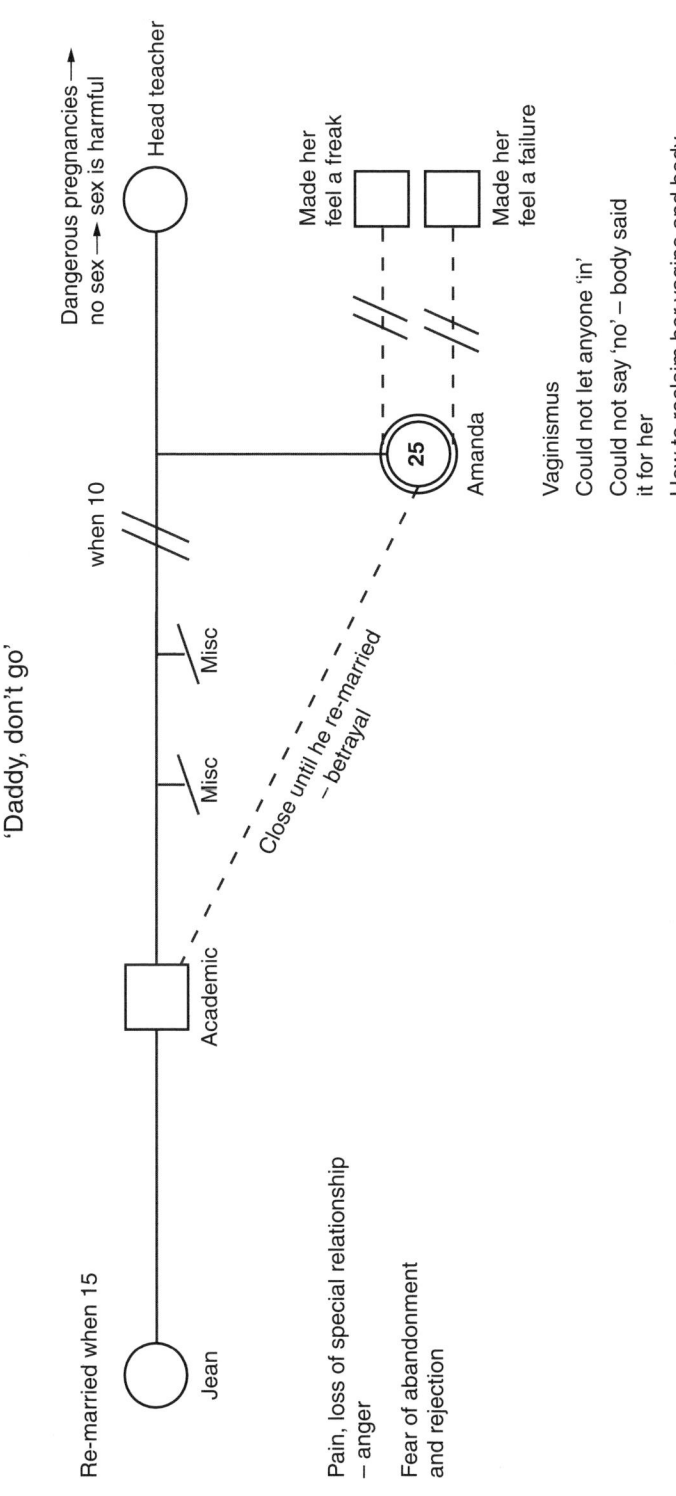

Figure 7.4 'Daddy, don't go.'

Her parents had divorced when she was ten, but Amanda was still daddy's girl until he met Jean, four years later. Jean and Amanda's father were having sex. Amanda felt betrayed: he was being 'unfaithful' to her. When they got married a year later, Amanda was so angry and jealous that she refused to go to the wedding and cut herself off from her father. She blamed him for the loss of their special relationship. Sex was not only dangerous, it was also destructive. Amanda carried on in a lonely cocoon, avoiding relationships, but safe from pain and rejection.

Amanda needed to reclaim her body as an adult and forgive her father for abandoning her. She also needed to understand what her mother's experience had been like and know that she did not have to repeat it.

I suggested she see a gynaecologist for reassurance. We worked with self-focus exercises until Amanda felt comfortable with her genitals and was able to introduce a finger into her vagina.

Soon after, Amanda contacted her father and arranged to meet him. She did not have a boyfriend yet, but she felt much more able to have a relationship and was looking forward to sharing a positive sexual experience.

■ Both partners

■ Loss of desire

Loss of desire is probably the most common sexual problem and affects both men and women.

Definition: Deficient or absent sexual fantasies and desire for sexual activity – also known as hypoactive sexual desire disorder or inhibited sexual desire.

What is desire?
- A thought.
- Feeling.
- Sensation.
- Instinct.
- Drive.
- Appetite.
- Need.

It is:

- psychological
- emotional
- physiological
- biological
- hormonal
- neurological
- evolutional.

Desire involves communication and feedback between body and mind, both conscious and unconscious. Any breakdown in the system at any point will affect desire.

It is important to acknowledge that there is a wide range of levels of libido and that accepting difference is part of the couple's work.

Desire will also be affected by the following factors.

1. • Illness.
   • Trauma.
   • Injury.
   • Medical and gynaecological procedures.
   • Medication.
   • Contraception.
   • Addiction.
2. • Pregnancy, childbirth and breast-feeding.
   • Affairs.
   • Work problems.
   • Family problems.
   • Bereavement.
   • Loss.
   • Crises.
3. • Depression.
   • Stress.
   • Anger.
   • Anxiety.
   • Fear.
   • Guilt.
   • Shame.
   • Low self-esteem.
4. • Negative experience of sex.
   • Sexual identity issues.
   • Body image.
   • Cultural and religious issues.
   • Partner dysfunction.
   • Relationship problems.
5. • Moving from 'in love' to 'loving'.
   • Unresolved Oedipal issues.
   • Mother/Madonna/whore split.
   • Fear of intimacy and commitment.
   • Fear of losing control.
   • Unconscious conflicts.

In the context of the relationship, loss of desire may be a powerful way of expressing anger and resentment. In this particular power struggle, the person who does not want sex holds the power and is punishing their partner, whether consciously or unconsciously.

Anxiety, whether sexual or other, will lead to avoidance and repression as defences.

Survivors of sexual abuse may have loss of desire because they have been used and manipulated in situations where they have had no control. Sex is experienced as threatening and unsafe. Sexual abandonment entails trust and vulnerability. It may feel safer to shut down one's desire than to risk the dangers of sex and the temporary loss of self.

When one has failed to make a real separation from the opposite-sex parent, sex may unconsciously be associated with incest. The taboo on sex is then projected onto the partner who is seen as a non-sexual being.

Lack of time appears to be a major reason for loss of desire. People lead such busy and stressful lives that sex is no longer prioritised. Couples who live together with equal gender roles end up like flat-mates or siblings. There is no gender differentiation. They have lost touch with their evolutionary drive.

Moving from the honeymoon 'in love' phase to the 'loving' phase affects desire. One's high expectations can no longer be met, the loss of excitement is not tolerated, and the partner is no longer experienced as a sexual being. 'I don't fancy her/him any more' and 'The spark has gone' are the two most common complaints.

Given all the possibilities for loss of desire, the therapist will have ample material to explore and issues to address.

Desire is a subtle and complex phenomenon that can be affected by a wide range of factors.

Sometimes one needs to remember that although the sexual urge is instinctive, making love is learned.

■ Sensate focus

Sensate focus is the most widely used technique in sex therapy and is used to treat all of the sexual dysfunctions. It was pioneered by Masters and Johnson in the United States in 1966. It is also extremely useful as a diagnostic tool, both physical and psychological.

Sensate focus is a de-sensitisation and gradual exposure process, involving a series of exercises that the couple agree to do on a regular basis at home and discuss afterwards with the therapist.

Teaching a couple how to make love again is entering a very delicate and personal area of their lives. This work is directive. The therapist needs to feel comfortable about giving instructions and do so with clarity and sensitivity at all times. She is taking on the role of educator, and needs to be confident and consistent, positive and encouraging. The exercises may appear to be artificial and lacking in spontaneity. The couple may feel nervous and embarrassed, resistant and defensive. There needs to be a strong therapeutic alliance based on trust and respect. Working with humour can defuse anxiety.

The first step is to check any physical causes for the dysfunction and put the situation in the context of the couple's life stage.

Relationship issues need exploring. The couple have to be motivated enough to make a commitment to each other and to the therapy in terms of time and application. The process usually takes a minimum of three months.

The therapist is negotiating a contract with the couple. They are negotiating one with each other. The therapist has to provide good modelling with firm boundaries and leave no area of doubt as far as the instructions for the exercises go.

Sensate focus is literally about getting back in touch with the senses, focusing on touch, sight, smell, taste and sound. It is sensual, not sexual. There is no goal, no pressure, no expectation, no need to perform, no right or wrong. The emphasis is on getting in touch with sensations and feelings, and discovering what it is like to become close and intimate again. It is more about being than doing. Arousal is incidental.

Each partner will give the other equal time and attention, equal giving and receiving, equal responsibility.

The first rule of sensate focus is for the couple to agree not to have sexual intercourse for the foreseeable future.

Some couples will say that they are not having intercourse anyway. The difference is that this is an agreed contract between them. The ban on intercourse removes any pressure from, and expectation of, sex. It can be very liberating for the couple because they can have physical contact without fear of having to perform.

Through the exercises the couple are given permission to learn what gives them pleasure before giving pleasure to their partner.

It is a process that removes a major source of anxiety, helps to build trust and improves the level of communication.

■ Sensate Focus 1 (SF1)

- The couple will be asked to carry out this exercise two or three times a week.
- They need to put aside one hour during which they will not be interrupted.
- They need to be in a private, warm, comfortable place (which is not necessarily the bedroom and its association with failure).
- There can be cushions, candles, music, a glass of wine, oil or talc, etc.
- Repeat the ban on intercourse and the rationale.
- Ask them to shower or bathe first and to lie down together naked with some light in the room.
- They are going to take it in turns to touch, stroke and caress each other from top to toe, first the back of the body, then the front, from head to foot without touching the genitals, buttocks or breasts.
- SF1 is for the giver, not the receiver. It is about rediscovering what it feels like to touch one's partner in an intimate and sensual way. It is not about turning the partner on.
- The giver can experiment with different types of touch, experience the different skin textures, explore unfamiliar parts of the body.
- The receiver may ask the giver to stop if she/he experiences anything uncomfortable or unpleasant.
- When the first person has completed the task (20–30 minutes) the partners change over.
- It is essential that the partners have an equal amount of time.
- If there is any sexual arousal on either side, it should be acknowledged, but nothing needs to be done about it.
- If the person experiences a desire to masturbate this can be done alone afterwards.
- Ask the couple to repeat the instructions back so that there are no misunderstandings.
- Ask them to choose who goes first. The giver is responsible for setting the time and place for the exercise.

- Explain that you will be asking for specific and detailed feedback at the following session.

Feedback on SF1
Ask the following questions.

- Who organised and initiated the session?
- How many times did they do the exercise?
- What was their overall experience of the exercise?
- How did it feel to be touching?
- How did it feel to be touched?
- What felt good; what felt not so good?
- Were they able to focus?
- What were they thinking?
- Was it easier giving or receiving?
- Did they talk to each other during or after the exercise?
- What did they learn about themselves?
- What did they learn about their partner?
- If they did the exercise more than once, were the sessions different?
- In what way?
- Ask them about their thoughts, feelings, sensations and fantasies.
- Check for assumptions.
- Reframe any negative perceptions.
- Give reassurance, affirmation, reinforcement and encouragement.

The therapist needs to work with the information she is being given by each partner and at the same time be aware of the interaction in the room, which will reflect their unconscious feelings.

Avoidance, blocks and defences are symptomatic of anger, anxiety, guilt, shame, inhibition, fear of intimacy, fear of rejection, lack of trust, power struggle and conflict.

Encourage them to express their feelings in the here and now.

Sometimes the couple will not co-operate enough to set up a first session, or one will sabotage the process from the start.

Some couples will not trust themselves or their partner to lie naked together. Suggest they wear nightgowns or underwear and just lie next to each other holding hands. This may be the most intimacy they can manage.

Either partner may be put back in touch with negative experiences of sex, abuse or violence that they may never have talked about.

These are only some of the issues that may arise from the experience of sensate focus. The therapist needs to be able to respond to the problems as they arise and work with both the conscious and the unconscious issues.

The exercise is to be repeated on at least three separate occasions or more until both partners are completely confident and comfortable with it.

■ Sensate Focus 2 (SF2)

SF2 is exactly the same as SF1 only this time the breasts, buttocks and genitals are included.

It is still primarily a sensual exercise with no sexual goal. It is still about the giver exploring the partner's body without any intention of giving pleasure. The receiver may feel pleasure and desire, he may have an erection, she may lubricate. This can be acknowledged, but nothing overtly sexual is done about it.

This phase is known as 'SF2 non-demand'.

It enables the couple to get back in touch with each other's whole body in a sensual, non-demanding way.

It also shows them that arousal and desire can occur spontaneously without being strived for.

If either partner is reluctant to do the exercise they can go back to SF1 and discuss the problems with the therapist. When the couple feel ready to move on, they can proceed to the next exercise, which is called 'SF2 demand'.

This is the first time that they are going to focus on giving their partner pleasure, starting with SF1 and asking each other for what they would each like. Having found out what gives oneself pleasure, one now focuses on what gives the partner pleasure.

There is still no goal for orgasm, even though it may occur from mutual stimulation. It is at this point that many couples will break the 'no intercourse' rule and find themselves agreeing to make love. This is fine as long as there has been no pressure on either side.

Like the previous exercise, this exercise is repeated until both partners feel good about it. Any time there is a block, they need to go back to SF1 and start again.

■ Sensate Focus 3 (SF3)

SF3 is stop/start vaginal containment and is particularly helpful for the male dysfunctions. After SF1 and SF2, the man lies on his back and the woman is on top. She stimulates him until he is erect, and he inserts the tip of his penis into her vagina. There is no movement. This is repeated several times.

Again, it is possible that the ban on intercourse will be broken.

■ Sensate Focus 4 (SF4)

SF4 is the same as SF3 but with movement.

■ Overview

Working with SF1 and SF2 and exploring the resistances will usually be extremely effective for most couples, especially those presenting with loss of desire, because it offers them the chance to break old habits and find the trust and intimacy they have lost.

Sometimes just a temporary ban on intercourse is liberating enough for a couple to get back in touch with each other physically and emotionally, so that they can go from no sex to good sex with a deeper understanding about giving and receiving pleasure.

Example: 'The danger of sex'

Andrew and Alice wanted to have a baby, but she had suffered loss of desire since they had got married two years previously. (*See* Figure 7.5.)

They were having sex very occasionally but she felt angry. He had stopped initiating because he did not want to be rejected.

Andrew was caring and supportive, and very devoted. He had Alice on a pedestal. Alice was volatile and emotional. She was attracted by Andrew's creativity, which she found quite exciting compared to her dry legal world. Andrew found her warm and open, in contrast to his family.

Their sexual relationship was satisfactory at first. They lived together for a year before getting married, which was a joint decision.

After they married Alice turned 30 and felt older and less attractive. Sex became perfunctory. She admitted to a fear of commitment. Andrew described their sex life as routine, not very adventurous. Alice said she found it difficult to let go and became more and more restrictive: missionary position only.

Her previous relationships had been short-lived; she had had lots of flings and one-night stands. Sex had been exciting and gratifying. But she felt very ambivalent with Andrew. Married sex was not supposed to be raunchy, yet she wanted him to be more assertive. He understandably felt confused. Sex for him was about intimacy and bonding.

When we looked at their genogram we found a lot of useful information.

Andrew's family were polite and formal. Anger was never expressed; sex was never discussed. Andrew had had a holiday fling which had resulted in a son, whom he had never seen and had no contact with. He needed to mourn that loss.

Alice's family were expressive and argumentative. She described her father as open and creative, but her mother was emotional and manipulative. She was afraid she was like her. Her parents had married because her mother was pregnant. They had split up, got back together, had an unplanned baby, who was ten years younger than Alice, and had split up again.

Both Andrew and Alice's experience was that sex led to unwanted pregnancies and trouble. Consciously they wanted a baby, but unconsciously they were afraid.

Alice had no experience of sex with intimacy but felt guilty about enjoying married sex. She was professionally ambitious and successful and was disappointed by Andrew's laid-back attitude to work – and to sex. Andrew was no longer initiating or responding.

When I explained the sensate focus programme they seemed keen. But they were half an hour late the following session, which delayed the implementation of SF1 and was proof of their anxiety.

She managed to initiate the exercises two sessions later. It went fine but what came out of it was that there were gender issues. She was driven but wanted him to be more macho. He gave her emotional stability but was not allowed to be sexy. She was too dominating; he felt emasculated.

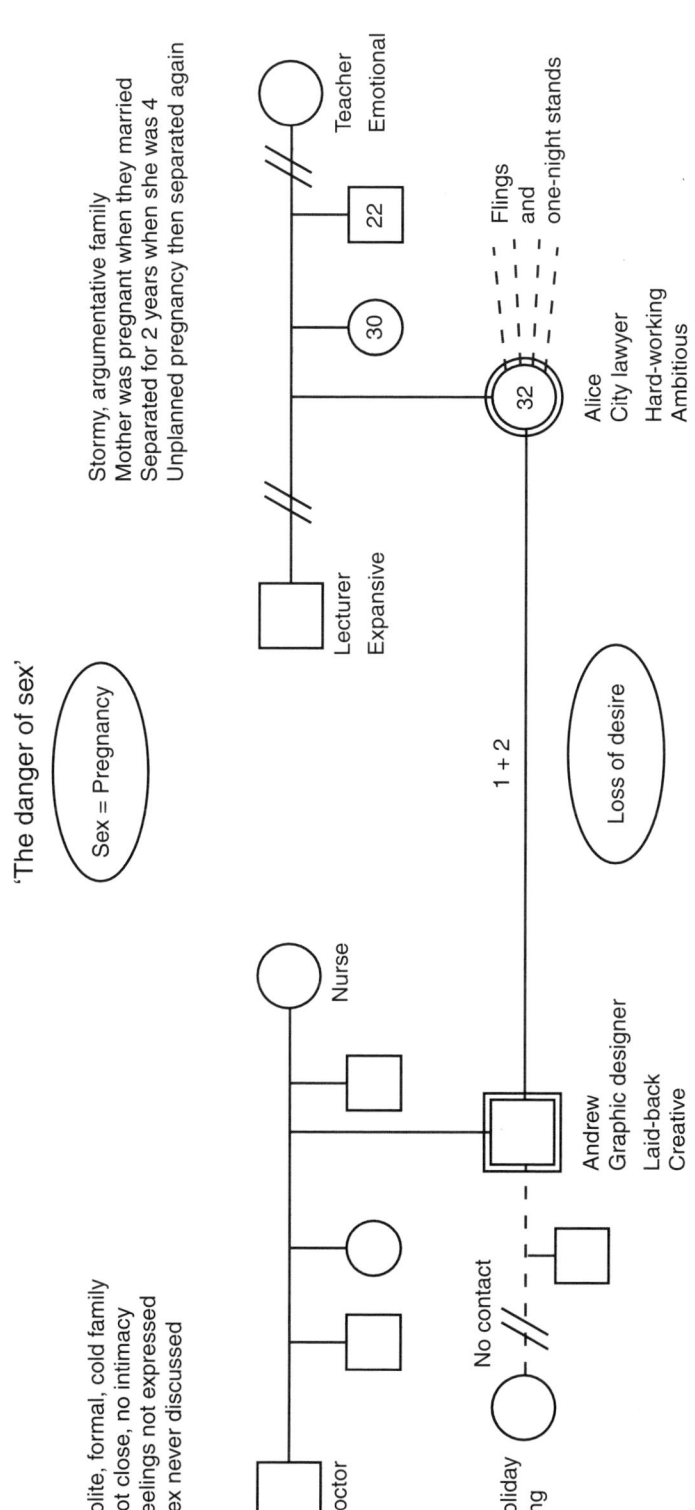

'The danger of sex'

Sex = Pregnancy

Stormy, argumentative family
Mother was pregnant when they married
Separated for 2 years when she was 4
Unplanned pregnancy then separated again

Teacher
Emotional

Lecturer
Expansive

Flings
and
one-night stands

Alice
City lawyer
Hard-working
Ambitious

Loss of desire

1 + 2

Polite, formal, cold family
Not close, no intimacy
Feelings not expressed
Sex never discussed

Nurse

Doctor

No contact

Holiday
fling

Andrew
Graphic designer
Laid-back
Creative

Figure 7.5 'The danger of sex.'

SF1 gave them equality and confidence. They were able to communicate about their assumptions and expectations. Somehow they could not find time to do the SF2 exercises. We discussed their anxieties. Both of them found it too artificial.

After doing 'SF2 demand' once, they broke the rules and had sex, which was her idea. He was thrilled, but she got scared and backed off again.

We went back to the beginning and started again. They got to the same point and had a huge row. They both felt hurt and angry and confused. Eventually he took responsibility for all the times he had rejected her. She carried the problem; he had to own his part in it.

Her loss of desire was a way of having control in the relationship, but it was also partly his projected fear and anxiety about commitment.

We agreed to stop the exercises and work on other aspects of the relationship. After four more sessions, Andrew and Alice were able to make love and were talking about trying for a baby. This time they meant it. I did not fully understand the transformation, but perhaps I did not need to.

Further reading

- Bancroft JH (1989) *Human Sexuality and its Problems*. Churchill Livingstone, London.
- Bass E (2002) *The Courage to Heal: a guide for women survivors of child sexual abuse*. Vermilion, London.
- Berman J and Berman L (2001) *For Women Only: a revolutionary guide to reclaiming your sex life*. Virago, London.
- Christopher E (1991) *Psychosexual Problems*. BACP, Rugby.
- Comfort A (2002) *The Joy of Sex*. 30th Anniversary Pocket Edition. Mitchell Beazley, London.
- Davies B and Perrett A (2000) *Psychodynamic Approaches to Sexual Problems*. Open University Press, Buckingham.
- Friday N (1979) *My Secret Garden*. Quartet Books, London.
- Godson S (2002) *The Sex Book*. Cassell, London.
- Gray J (2003) *Mars and Venus in the Bedroom: a guide to lasting romance and passion*. Vermilion, London.
- Hawton K (1985) *Sex Therapy: a practical guide*. Oxford University Press, Oxford.
- Heiman J and LoPiccolo J (1988) *Becoming Orgasmic: a sexual and personal growth programme for women*. Piatkus, London.
- Hooper A (1992) *The Body Electric: a unique account of sex therapy for women*. Pandora, London.
- Jehu D (1990) *Beyond Sexual Abuse: therapy with women who were childhood victims*. Wiley, Chichester.
- Kaplan H (1999) *The New Sex Therapy: active treatment of sexual dysfunctions*. Brunner Routledge, London.
- Kitzinger S (1985) *Women's Experience of Sex*. Penguin Books, London.
- Litvinoff S (1992) *The Relate Guide to Sex in Loving Relationships*. Vermilion, London.
- Scharff D (1988) *The Sexual Relationship: an object relations view of sex and the family*. Routledge, London.
- Schnarch D (1991) *Constructing the Sexual Crucible: an integration of sexual and marital therapy*. WW Norton, New York.
- Skrine R (1997) *Blocks and Freedoms in Sexual Life: a handbook of psychosexual medicine*. Radcliffe Medical Press, Oxford.
- Stoller R (1994) *Perversion: the erotic form of hatred*. Karnac Books, London.
- Storr A (1977) *Sexual Deviation*. Penguin, Harmondsworth.
- Zilbergeld B (1983) *Men and Sex*. HarperCollins, London.

CHAPTER 8

Conclusion

Working with couples is like playing in a mixed doubles tennis match when one is used to the longer rallies of one to one. One needs to think quickly, instinctively and intuitively, as well as countertransferentially. Understanding the action and reaction in the here and now is crucial – the therapist is observer, facilitator and interpreter of the relationship.

The essential elements of couples work can be summarised as follows.

From the psychodynamic angle one needs to understand the concepts of projective identification and unconscious collusive fit between the couple. A replay of Oedipal issues will also be present.

Systemically one needs to see where the relationship is in the context of family patterns and life stages. This is where genograms are particularly useful. One will be working with challenging the status quo and exploring change.

From a cognitive and behavioural point of view, one will help the clients to reframe, change old habits, set goals and complete tasks.

Psychosexual work starts with accurate and detailed information about physiology and the stages of desire and arousal. The clients' sexual relationship needs to be contextualised within their psychological development and current life stages.

There is a high incidence of incest and sexual abuse in its broadest sense among clients who present for psychosexual therapy. These painful issues can be helpfully addressed by the informed and sensitive therapist.

With so much information in the media about the techniques of sex and what to do when it goes wrong, fewer clients are presenting with the classic mechanical dysfunctions. But more and more are presenting with loss of desire – in particular couples in their thirties who seem to have it all, but have lost touch with their primitive sexual urges. The major causes are to be found in feelings of anger and anxiety, unresolved Oedipal issues and life crises, past and present. Lack of gender differentiation also plays a part.

Sensate focus is the single most useful diagnostic and problem-solving tool in psychosexual therapy and is accessible and available to all therapists.

Working with couples is a most satisfying and enriching experience. In a Winnicottian sense, the consulting room becomes a safe and creative place in which to explore and play with the very subtle and complex interchanges and feelings that make up a relationship between a couple. Still in the spirit of Winnicott, one does not need to be a highly qualified therapist in order to work with couples – one just needs to be 'good enough'.

Helpful resources

■ Professional practice

British Association for Counselling and Psychotherapy
1 Regent Place
Rugby CV21 2PJ
Tel: 01788 550899 Fax: 0870 443 5160
www.bac.co.uk
Promotes standards and services in counselling and training, nationally and internationally. Promotes information and advice on all matters related to counselling. It
also provides lists of accredited counsellors in local areas.

British Association for Sexual and Relationship Therapy (BASRT)
PO Box 13686
London SW20 9ZH
Tel/Fax: 020 8543 2707
www.basrt.org.uk
BASRT is concerned with sexual and relationship function. It provides therapy for
couples and accredits counsellors in sexual and relationship work. Members receive
Sexual and Relationship Therapy, an international quarterly academic journal.

The Child Psychotherapy Trust
Star House
104–108 Grafton Road
London NW5 4BD
Tel: 020 7284 1355
www.childpsychotherapytrust.org.uk
A charity that works to improve access to appropriate child psychotherapy of children
and families in need of help.

Institute of Family Therapy
24–32 Stephenson Way
London NW1 2HX
Tel: 020 7391 9150 Fax: 020 7391 9169
Best time to phone: 10.00am–5.00pm, Monday–Friday
www.instituteoffamilytherapy.org.uk
The Institute of Family Therapy acts as a resource for training professionals in family
therapy. There is also a clinical practice and the group welcomes self-referrals from
individuals or from other professionals. Fees are on a sliding scale depending on
income.

Jewish Marriage Council
23 Ravenshurst Avenue
London NW4 4EE
Tel: 020 8203 6311 Fax: 020 8203 8727
www.jmc-uk.org
An organisation providing counselling for anyone under stress or with a problem concerning relationships. It offers advice and group discussion for engaged and newly married couples.

London Marriage Guidance
76a New Cavendish Street
London W1G 9PE
Tel: 020 7580 1087 Fax: 020 7637 4546
www.londonmarriageguidance.org.uk
Individual and couple relationship counselling.

Marriage Care
1 Blythe Mews
Blythe Road
London W14 0NW
Tel: 020 7371 1341 Fax: 020 7371 4921
www.marriagecare.org.uk
Offers relationship counselling and preparation for marriage.

Marriage Care Scotland
10 Panmure Street
Dundee DD1 2BW
Tel: 01382 227551
Relationship counselling for couples and individuals, pre-marriage work and education work.

Muslim Marriage Guidance Council
8 Caburn Road
Hove
Sussex BN3 6EF
24-hour contact line: 07971 861972
A service to help cross-cultural marriages and provide counselling. It offers services in a wide range of languages.

NAFSIYAT
Inter-Cultural Therapy Centre
278 Seven Sisters Road
London N4 2HY
Tel: 020 7263 4130
E-mail: nafsiyat-therapy@supanet.com
NAFSIYAT provides psychotherapy by therapists from a wide range of ethnic and cultural backgrounds for clients, individuals, families and adolescents, from diverse backgrounds. A wide range of languages is also available.

Partner Therapy Group
Tel: 07977 493667
www.partnertherapy.com
A web-based advisory and self-referral service specialising in sexual and relationship problems. All practitioners are registered with the UK Council for Psychotherapy.

Relate (National Marriage Guidance)
Herbert Gray College
Little Church Street
Rugby CV21 3AP
Tel: 01788 573241
www.relate.org.uk
Offers counselling and individual relationship counselling through 100 local centres.

■ Counselling and couple support

Albany Trust
239 Balham High Road
London SW17 7BE
Tel: 020 8767 1827
Albany Trust is a charitable foundation providing one-to-one, couple and group counselling and psychotherapy, both short- and long-term. It specialises in psychosexual problems, sexual identity, sexual compulsion and gender identity. It also deals with issues arising from anxiety in relationships, bereavement and feelings of low self-worth.

African Caribbean Family Mediation Service
2–4 St John's Crescent
London SW9 7LZ
Tel: 020 7737 2366 Fax: 020 7733 0637
www.acfms.org
A south London-based service offering relationship counselling, child-focused mediation, a home/school mediation service and a counselling service for men.

Asian Family Counselling Service
Suite 51, Windmill Place
2–4 Windmill Lane
Southall UB2 4NJ
Tel/Fax: 020 8571 3933
E-mail: afcs99@hotmail.com
An organisation providing marriage preparation, marriage enrichment and counselling. It aims to advance education among people of Asian origin on all aspects of marriage and family relationships.

National Family Mediation
9 Tavistock Place
London WC1H 9SN
Tel: 020 7383 5993 Fax: 020 7383 5994
www.nfm.u-net.com

One Plus One Marriage and Partnership Research
The Wells
7–15 Rosebery Avenue
London EC1R 4SP
Tel: 020 7841 3660 Fax: 020 7841 3670
www.oneplusone.org.uk for links to Springboard, a membership scheme providing access to information and resources.
One Plus One works closely with other marriage and family support organisations and has developed ground-breaking training and resources for those working with couples and their families.

The Tavistock Marital Studies Institute
Tavistock Centre
120 Belsize Lane
London NW3 5BA
Tel: 020 7435 7111 Fax: 020 7435 1080
www.tmsi.org.uk
The Institute is internationally recognised as a world leader in the psychoanalytic understanding of the couple relationship. It offers couple therapy and engages in research, training and consultations to the wider voluntary, health and statutory fields.

Westminster Pastoral Foundation
23 Kensington Square
London W8 5HN
Tel: 020 7361 4864 Fax: 020 7361 4860
www.wpf.org.uk
WPF is a large charitable provider of general counselling and psychotherapy services and psychodynamic counselling and psychotherapy training.

Index